CHRONIC INFECTION, *CHLAMYDIA* AND CORONARY HEART DISEASE

Developments in Cardiovascular Medicine

VOLUME 218

The titles published in this series are listed at the end of this volume.

Chronic Infection, *Chlamydia* and Coronary Heart Disease

by

SANDEEP GUPTA MD, MRCP
Cardiological Sciences,
St George's Hospital Medical School,
London, U.K.

and

A. JOHN CAMM MD, FRCP
Cardiological Sciences,
St George's Hospital Medical School,
London, U.K.

KLUWER ACADEMIC PUBLISHERS
DORDRECHT / BOSTON / LONDON

A C.I.P. Catalogue record for this book is available from the Library of Congress

ISBN 0-7923-5797-3

Published by Kluwer Academic Publishers,
P.O. Box 17, 3300 AA Dordrecht, The Netherlands.

Sold and distributed in North, Central and South America
by Kluwer Academic Publishers,
101 Philip Drive, Norwell, MA 02061, U.S.A.

In all other countries, sold and distributed
by Kluwer Academic Publishers,
P.O. Box 322, 3300 AH Dordrecht, The Netherlands.

Printed on acid-free paper

Cover figure adapted from 'Gupta S. and Camm A.J., Chlamydia association or causation?.BMJ 1997; 314:1778-9' with permission.

Printed in the Netherlands.

Contents

Foreword

This is an original and timely book, which reviews the role of chronic infection (in particular, *Chlamydia pneumoniae*) in the genesis of coronary heart disease (CHD).

To a generation raised on the powerful epidemiological and trial evidence linking CHD to conventional risk factors, such as cigarette smoking, diet and lipids, and blood pressure, it may seem strange to contemplate antibiotics as a future cure. However, one only has to look at the field of gastroenterology to see how a novel hypothesis that *Helicobacter pylori* infection causes peptic ulceration led rapidly to major changes in treatment.

The book highlights a growing body of information which demonstrates that coronary and other arterial lesions contain *C. pneumoniae* (and other) microorganisms. The question as to whether these microorganisms are merely passengers, carried in by the phagocytes associated with plaques, or whether they are actually responsible for the inflammatory lesion, is under intense study. We also need to know whether or not these chronic infections are merely markers for social conditions, such as poverty or deprivation.

The authors – Sandeep Gupta and John Camm – are two leading investigators in this growing area of cardiovascular research. In this book, they synthesise the current position on 'Chronic infection, *Chlamydia* and CHD', and provide – for both newcomers to the field and those already within it – an opportunity to examine the main evidence to date and to ponder on areas of future research. Of course, many texts will follow with progression and developments of the 'infection hypothesis', but there is clearly a place for a concise, clearly-written and current review. The book provides this, focusing on the important observational and experimental data. Fascinating and difficult questions remain to be answered, but by the end of the text we are left with a feeling that exciting research lies ahead.

Peter Sleight MD DM FECP
Professor Emeritus of
Cardiovascular Medicine
John Radcliffe Hospital
Oxford, UK

Preface

We still have much to learn about the pathogenesis of coronary heart disease (CHD). Despite increasing understanding of the disease's causation and progression, and continuing advances in its prevention and treatment, CHD remains a major cause of human morbidity and mortality worldwide. Indeed, countries in eastern Europe and the developing world are currently experiencing an 'epidemic' of cardiovascular diseases. This situation contrasts with the falling CHD mortality rates seen in industrialised countries over the last 25 years. Further, the prevalence and postulated interactions of established, classical atherogenic risk factors fail to account for the wide variations in CHD prevalence and severity found from population to population. Such epidemiological findings mirror the common clinical experience of encountering individual patients with unequivocal evidence of severe coronary atheroma in the absence of factors such as cigarette smoking, hypertension, diabetes mellitus, hyperlipidaemia or family history of atherosclerotic disease.

These gaps in our knowledge about CHD have prompted a search for other potential (and hitherto unrecognised) influences on atherogenesis. In particular, interest has focused recently on the potential pathogenetic roles of common chronic infections and inflammation. This book aims to provide an overview of the various infective agents and inflammatory processes possibly implicated in aetiology and progression of atherosclerosis and CHD, concentrating on the organism for which evidence of direct involvement is strongest – *Chlamydia pneumoniae.*

Chapter 1 provides an outline of the epidemiology of atherosclerosis, proposed models of atherogenesis and the relevance of inflammation and its mediators in this setting. Evidence linking various infective organisms with atherosclerosis is reviewed in Chapter 2. Next, Chapter 3 then elaborates on the current knowledge of relevant microbiology of *C. pneumoniae*, and this information forms a background to discussion (in Chapter 4) of the mounting seroepidemiological and laboratory, pathological and clinical evidence suggesting that this organism is involved in the pathogenesis of atherosclerosis, and in particular, CHD. Chapter 5 considers potential mechanisms by which *C. pneumoniae* may contribute to atherogenesis (including potential interplay with established CHD risk factors). The results of relevant pilot antibiotic studies and the protocols for ongoing antibiotic intervention trials in CHD are detailed in Chapter 6. Finally, Chapter 7 offers a perspective on the putative role of *C. pneumoniae* in atherosclerosis, future lines of pertinent research and possible implications for management of patients with CHD.

S Gupta
AJ Camm

Acknowledgements

We are grateful to Juan Carlos Kaski, to whom we express a special acknowledgement. His background work and research on the mechanisms of atherogenesis and the link with inflammation set the foundation for exploring the role of *Chlamydia* and other infections in coronary heart disease, and has also inspired many other related research projects.

We also express our gratitude to the British Heart Foundation, which has been instrumental in the financial support of research in our institution, in particular on the work on 'infection, inflammation and coronary heart disease'.

We are most thankful to the team at PPSI, UK, who helped in the editing and layout of the book. Finally, we are grateful to Nettie Dekker at Kluwer Academic Publishers for publishing our work.

List of Figures

List of Tables

Chapter 1: Atherosclerosis and coronary heart disease

Introduction

Atherosclerotic vascular disease, in particular, coronary heart disease (CHD), is a major cause of human morbidity and mortality in both industrialised and developing countries. In the UK, for example, nearly 170,000 people die each year as a result of CHD (25% of all deaths).[1] Similarly, in the USA, CHD causes around 700,000 (40% of) deaths each year.[2,3] However, there are very wide variations in the incidence of CHD worldwide. For instance, data from the World Health Organization (WHO) MONItoring of trends and determinants in CArdiovascular disease (MONICA) study assessing CHD and risk factors in 38 populations from 21 countries show that age-standardised annual cardiovascular event (fatal and non-fatal) rates (during 1985–1987) in men ranged from 76/100,000 in Beijing, China to 915/100,000 in North Karelia, Finland, and in women, from 30/100,000 in Catalonia, Spain to 256/100,000 in Glasgow, UK.[4] Also, while CHD mortality rates in many industrialised countries have fallen over the past 20–30 years (e.g. by 50–60% in Australia, Canada, Japan and the USA), there have been striking increases in the rates in eastern/central Europe (e.g. 25–35% rises in Romania and Poland) and in developing countries.

Classical risk factors: An inadequate explanation

Classical atherogenic risk factors include: cigarette smoking, hypercholesterolaemia, diabetes mellitus, hypertension and a positive family history of CHD. Such factors are important for predicting total (absolute) CHD risk in individual patients. However, variations in the presence or severity of these factors probably account for no more than half of the known differences in prevalence and severity of CHD.[5,6] In addition, up to 30% of patients presenting with myocardial infarction (MI) have none of these risk factors.[7] Furthermore, in some populations, the marked frequency of classical risk factors is not associated with a high prevalence of CHD.[8] One example of this is the so-called 'French paradox'.[9] Moderate, widespread consumption of certain types of alcohol helps protect the French population against CHD (possibly via anti-oxidant effects), despite a relatively high rate of cigarette smoking among such people. Similarly, the Japanese have very high smoking rates but, nevertheless, very low CHD mortality rates and high life expectancy. Furthermore, Pima Indians have the highest rates of obesity and diabetes mellitus in the world but, even so, rarely develop CHD. Yet another apparent discrepancy is the low prevalence of CHD among African–Caribbean populations despite particularly high prevalence rates of diabetes mellitus, hypertension and cerebrovascular disease.[10]

So why the variations?

These hitherto unexplained epidemiological anomalies have prompted speculation about, and research into, other potential influences on the aetiology and progression of atherosclerosis. Such factors include:

- 'Programming' in fetal life as a result of maternal malnutrition ('Barker's hypothesis').[11] Small size at birth is associated with several coronary risk factors including: high blood pressure, non-insulin-dependent diabetes mellitus and high plasma fibrinogen levels. The findings have led to the hypothesis that later development of CHD is programmed *in utero*, with fetal responses to undernutrition leading to persisting changes in metabolism and organ structure.
- The 'insulin-resistance syndrome'. This comprises clustering of pre-atherogenic factors, such as central obesity, hyperinsulinaemia and hypertriglyceridaemia, which may interact and predispose to premature CHD.[12]
- Defects in homocysteine metabolism that may lead to an increased thrombotic tendency.[13] Evidence suggests that homocysteine may affect the coagulation system and the resistance of the endothelium to thrombosis, and perhaps also interfere with the vasodilator and anti-thrombotic functions of nitric oxide.[14]

Several prospective, nested case–control studies have found a relation between total homocysteine levels and frequency of vascular disease. A single study has also confirmed that serum total homocysteine levels are a strong predictor of mortality in patients with angiographically confirmed CHD.[15]

- Defined and as yet unidentified genetic factors (including variability of plasma lipoprotein(a) in normal populations and apolipoprotein E polymorphism).[16,17]

Defining whether, and to what extent, such mechanisms play a role in atherothrombosis requires further investigation.

Chronic infection is the other major factor implicated increasingly in the pathogenesis of atherosclerosis.[18] However, before considering the detailed evidence suggesting such a relationship between chronic infection and CHD, it is worth reviewing briefly atherosclerosis itself. An exhaustive discussion of the classical (and more modern) hypotheses on, and established facts about, this complex condition is beyond the intended scope of this book. Instead, we concentrate on features of atherogenesis that indicate a pivotal contributory role for chronic inflammation and, potentially, therefore, chronic infection.

What is atherosclerosis?

Atherosclerosis is the sequence of changes that produces focal obstructions (atherosclerotic plaques) in the endothelium of large and medium-sized arteries. Characteristic processes in the formation and subsequent development of such plaques include: accumulation of cholesterol-rich material in the endothelium (atherosis); the expansion of fibrous tissue (sclerosis); and inflammation that involves monocytes, macrophages and T-lymphocytes. When the bulk of plaque tissue reduces the luminal diameter of an affected vessel by more than about 70%, blood flow is compromised significantly. This may lead to clinical manifestations of atherosclerotic disease, such as angina or intermittent claudication. Disruption of a vulnerable or unstable plaque with a subsequent change in plaque geometry and thrombosis, may result in acute, partial or complete occlusion of the affected vessel leading to the clinical manifestations of acute coronary syndromes, such as MI or unstable angina (see Figure 1).[19,20]

Figure 1: Stages of atherogenesis

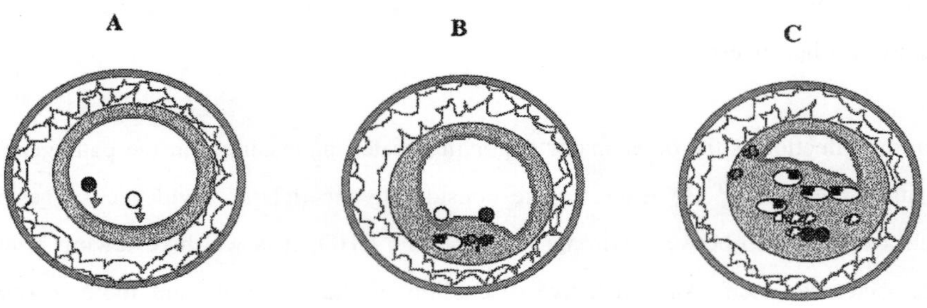

Schematic section through a coronary artery. Injury to the endothelium (e.g. caused by toxins, low-density lipoprotein [LDL], bacteria, viruses) leads to increased vascular permeability and attachment and migration of monocytes (**A**). Subsequent accumulation of intracellular lipid and foam cell formation occur (**B**). Activated monocytes, platelets and other cells secrete growth factors, triggering smooth muscle proliferation in the subendothelial space. The lesion matures to form a fibrous plaque comprising an inflammatory cell infiltrate, collagen, lipids and calcium (**C**). Erosion and eventual rupture of the fibrous cap may trigger formation of superimposed thrombus.

Variable plaque development

The lipid accumulation, cell proliferation and synthesis of extracellular matrix which comprise atherogenesis do not follow a predictable course. New, seemingly advanced lesions often become apparent in coronary segments that were angiographically normal only months earlier. Also, clinical evidence indicates that arteries with the most severe stenoses are not necessarily the vessels most likely to go on to occlude. Indeed, mildly stenosed coronary lesions may be associated with significant progression to severe stenosis or total occlusion, and may account for up to two-thirds of cases of patients presenting with acute coronary syndromes.[19]

Classical hypotheses of atherogenesis

Early ideas

Hypotheses on the pathogenesis of atherosclerosis were suggested originally by Rokitansky in 1852,[21] Virchow in 1856[22] and Duguid in 1946.[23] Virchow proposed that minor arterial wall injury resulted in an inflammatory response, leading to accumulation of plasma constituents within the intima of the artery. Rokitansky's belief (subsequently elaborated by Duguid) was that encrustrations of small mural thrombi developed at sites of arterial injury and became organised as a result of growth of smooth muscle cells into them.[21] It was proposed that the resulting complexes became incorporated into the atheromatous lesions, and so helped further the progression of such lesions.

The monoclonal hypothesis

The monoclonal hypothesis, formulated in 1973, suggests that atherosclerotic lesions are a form of benign neoplasia.[24] It assumes that each lesion is derived from a single smooth muscle cell – the precursor of all other cells in a proliferating clone. This idea is based on the observation that in people who are heterozygous for isoenzymes of glucose 6-phosphate dehydrogenase (and whose cells might, therefore, be expected to contain equal quantities of these two isoenzymes), smooth muscle cells within atherosclerotic lesions express only one of the two isoforms. A later development of this notion suggests that each atherosclerotic lesion is a benign neoplasm derived from a cell that has been transformed by viruses, chemicals or other mutagens.

The 'response-to-injury' hypothesis

In 1973, the hypotheses on atherogenesis were combined with emerging knowledge of the biology of the arterial wall to generate the 'response-to-injury' model of atherosclerosis.[25] This concept has been modified in light of increased understanding of the interactions between blood and arterial cells, and of the role of cardiovascular risk factors in atherogenesis and endothelial cell disruption.[26] It has become the most widely accepted theory of atherosclerosis, and best fits with established facts about the disease. The model is discussed more fully in the next section.

The endothelium and its response to injury

The normal endothelium

The endothelium is a monolayer of elongated cells that lines all blood vessels. Healthy endothelium performs several regulatory and anti-atherosclerotic functions.[27] These include: local production of heparans, tissue plasminogen activator, thromboxane and thrombomodulin, as well as the continuous generation of nitric oxide; all of these elements help to maintain an anticoagulant surface and a state of so-called 'defensive' vasodilation. The endothelial cell layer also inhibits the adhesion and migration of inflammatory cells, limits growth and migration of smooth muscle cells and produces a limited proportion of the tissue matrix present in the intima.

Injury and atherosclerosis

How damage occurs

The 'response-to-injury' hypothesis of atherosclerosis states that endothelial cells at specific sites of low shear stress in the artery wall incur some form of 'injury'.[28] Inflammatory processes may both initiate and perpetuate such damage. Other influences may also compound the vascular injury. Such factors include: arterial hypertension, low-density-lipoprotein (LDL) cholesterol, glycosylated end-products, toxins in tobacco smoke, immune complexes, homocysteine and infection. Three types of arterial injury are described in this model. In type I injury, there is functional alteration of endothelial cells with no significant morphological change. In type II injury, part of the endothelium is denuded. Disruption of both the intima and media of the artery is present in type III injury.

Early plaque development

Endothelial cell damage is followed by development of the typical atherosclerotic plaque. This involves an increase in vascular permeability to lipids and monocytes/macrophages, together with migration and proliferation of smooth muscle cells. Endothelial dysfunction is regarded as a crucial, early event in the pathogenesis of atherosclerosis. This abnormal function usually manifests as increased accumulation of lipoprotein in the wall and the appearance of specific adhesive glycoproteins on the surface of the endothelial cells. In addition, monocytes and T-lymphocytes attach to the altered endothelium and migrate between its constituent cells under the influence of growth-regulatory molecules and chemoattractants. These chemical factors may be released locally by the altered endothelium, its adherent leucocytes and, possibly, underlying smooth muscle cells.[29,30]

As the atherogenic process continues, migrating cells penetrate further beneath the arterial surface, and the monocytes transform into tissue macrophages. Such macrophages can internalise oxidised cholesterol-containing LDLs (although not native unoxidised LDL).[31] The resulting accumulation of intracellular cholesterol esters transforms macrophages into foam cells. Together with accompanying lymphocytes, these foam cells make up the fatty streak, the characteristic lesion of early atheroma.[32-34] Such precursor lesions are commonly demonstrable in young people. For example, an autopsy study by Berenson *et al.* demonstrated atherosclerotic changes of the aortas and coronary arteries in persons aged 6–30 years.[35]

Formation of fibrous plaque

As atherogenesis progresses, smooth muscle cells in the endothelium proliferate, with formation of a connective tissue matrix comprising elastic fibre proteins, collagen and proteoglycans. This matrix eventually leads to the generation of a more advanced atherosclerotic lesion and, ultimately, to the establishment of a fibrous plaque and cap (see Figure 1).[28,32,36,37]

Relevant cell and mediator interactions

During the development of atherosclerotic plaques, the inflammatory cells recruited and resident in the lesions become 'activated',[38] and so produce growth factors such as platelet-derived growth factor-β (PDGF-β), fibroblast growth factor and heparan-like glycosaminoglycans. While tissue factor is expressed in excess (by macrophages and smooth muscle cells), locally generated cytokines (such as interleukin-1 [IL-1], interleukin-6 [IL-6] and monocyte chemoattractant protein-1) serve to amplify further the inflammatory and proliferative processes. In addition to their role in cholesterol metabolism in atherosclerotic lesions, activated macrophages increase platelet adhesion, secrete growth factors (including transforming growth factor-β [TGF-β][39] and PDGF-β[40]), all of which stimulate the activity of smooth muscle cells that are cytotoxic to neighbouring cells.[41] The monocyte surface forms an assembly plant for several adhesion proteins (such as CD11b and CD11c).[42] These surface integrin proteins (see page 13) may be upregulated by cytokines such as tissue necrosis factor-α (TNF-α), IL-1 or bacterial lipopolysaccharide (LPS).[43,44]

T-lymphocytes are present at all stages of atheroma, often in close association with macrophages,[45] and represent up to 20% of the cells present in fatty streaks and fibrous caps.[46] They are activated by major histocompatibility complex (MHC) proteins of antigen-presenting cells (i.e. endothelial cells or macrophages expressing HLA, HLA-DR antigens). The T-lymphocytes may be stimulated by oxidised LDL to produce interferon-γ, which both initiates cell proliferation and reduces cholesterol accumulation.[43] The lymphocytes, which predominate at the lateral edges of lesions,[47] may also be stimulated by modified lipoproteins, elements from the necrotic core of plaques, heat-shock proteins or viral proteins. Cytokines and other growth factors are similarly involved at several stages of atherogenesis, including: surface expression of adhesion molecules on endothelium; recruitment and activation of monocytes/macrophages and T-lymphocytes; regulation of smooth muscle growth and extracellular matrix formation; and induction of class II MHC molecules on antigen-presenting cells.[43–46,48]

Acute inflammation and plaque activity

Traditionally, coronary artery atheromatous lesions have been classified according to the extent to which they narrow the arterial lumen. However, from a pathophysiological perspective, such lesions may be described better as either 'inactive' or 'active'.[38] The transformation of an inactive plaque to an active one involves development of an acute inflammatory response within the lesions. This acute inflammatory component of atherogenesis has adverse effects both within the atherosclerotic plaque and on other parts of the coronary artery. For instance, activation of monocytes and macrophages in the plaque results in the release of cytokines and chemotactic factors that recruit other leucocytes to the lesion. Monocytes also release degradative enzymes such as the metalloproteinases; these enzymes break down connective tissue and can undermine the structural integrity of the plaque, leading to weakening and eventual rupture of the fibrous cap. Individual plaques can vary markedly with regard to their susceptibility to surface erosion and rupture, and their resultant thrombogenic potential. Plaques at highest risk of rupturing include those with activated and dysfunctional endothelium, a large lipid core with a thin fibrous cap, markedly increased amounts of tissue factor, and an abundance of inflammatory cells (including macrophages and T-lymphocytes).[49]

By synthesizing the procoagulant, tissue factor, monocytes and macrophages contribute directly to the thrombosis that follows plaque rupture. Procoagulant activity is also stimulated by activated lymphocytes, certain cytokines and bacterial LPS. Within the coronary artery lumen, elastase, collagenase, oxygen free radicals, leukotrienes and other substances secreted by activated granulocytes and monocytes further disrupt the plaque. These substances also depress myocardial function, exacerbate vasospasm and damage endothelium, both structurally and functionally. The functional loss of the endothelium increases the likelihood of vasoconstriction and thrombosis. Substances derived from leucocytes may also stimulate platelet aggregation, and products of platelet activation can promote neutrophil accumulation within the plaque.

Cells, mediators and CHD risk

As discussed above, central features of atherosclerosis include the recruitment and activation of various contributing cells and production of several local and systemic procoagulant and inflammatory mediators. The evidence linking such changes in cells and mediators with CHD and plausible roles for them in atherogenesis are discussed below.

Leucocytes and monocytes

White cell count and CHD

Several case–control and prospective studies have shown an association between the total blood leucocyte count and CHD.[50–53] In the Multiple Risk Factor Intervention Trial (MRFIT), total leucocyte count was significantly related to risk of having CHD.[54] Furthermore, a decrease in blood leucocyte count (from baseline level to that at the annual examination just prior to the cardiovascular event) was associated with a significant reduction in the risk of experiencing a future cardiovascular event. Although the leucocyte count is generally higher in cigarette smokers, the reported association of raised counts with CHD has usually appeared to be independent of smoking status.[50,53,54] There is some evidence that the band neutrophil count is an even better predictor of CHD than is the total leucocyte count.[55]

There are several mechanisms by which leucocytes could contribute directly to atherosclerosis.[56] For example, such cells tend to aggregate and embolise to microvessels under low-flow conditions.[57] Also, blood leucocytes may alter rheologic characteristics or cause endothelial injury and inflammation through the release of activated substances such as free radicals, long-acting oxidants, proteolytic enzymes and arachidonic acid metabolites.[58,59]

Monocyte count and CHD

Studies have demonstrated an association between the absolute monocyte count and CHD. Prentice *et al.* showed that monocyte (and neutrophil and eosinophil) counts were predictive of prevalent CHD, although cigarette smoking was not taken into account in their study.[60] In the Paris Prospective Study, Olivares *et al.* found a significant correlation between higher monocyte counts and raised incidences of MI and sudden coronary death, associations that were independent of patient age and smoking status.[61]

C-reactive protein

Increased circulating levels of acute phase reactants occur in most forms of inflammation, infection and tissue damage.[62] These reactants are produced primarily by hepatocytes following stimulation by cytokines secreted by activated macrophages. C-reactive protein (CRP) is an acute phase protein that amplifies the underlying cytokine stimulus of acute phase protein production. The plasma concentration of CRP is a reliable indicator of the overall level of inflammatory activity present in the body.[63]

Prediction in established atherosclerotic disease

Concentrations of CRP correlate directly with the presence and severity of coronary, cerebral and peripheral atherosclerosis.[64] For example, Luizzo and colleagues reported that, in patients admitted to hospital with unstable angina, an initial plasma concentration of CRP above 3mg/L (the 90th centile of the normal CRP distribution) was associated with a particularly poor clinical outcome, even in the absence of other evidence of more severe CHD.[65] Furthermore, in an investigation of 2121 patients with stable or unstable angina entered into the European Concerted Action on Thrombosis and disabilities (ECAT) study, those with CRP concentrations in the fifth quintile (i.e. above 3.6mg/L) had a twofold increased risk of developing further coronary events during a 2-year follow-up period.[66] This study provided the first evidence that CRP could predict clinical outcome in patients with stable angina; its authors speculated (as had other investigators) that raised CRP levels may reflect underlying inflammation or infection caused by organisms linked with atherosclerosis, such as *Chlamydia pneumoniae*[67] or *Helicobacter pylori.*[68]

Prediction of first atherosclerotic events

C-reactive protein levels can also indicate the likelihood of future CHD events in those without clinically overt atherosclerotic disease. Evidence for this comes from a 8-year prospective study conducted by Ridker *et al.*, in which the risk of developing a first thrombotic cardiovascular event was assessed in 543 apparently healthy men.[69] Baseline plasma CRP concentrations were higher in men who went on to have MIs or ischaemic strokes (threefold higher relative risk for men in the quartile of highest CRP levels; $p<0.001$). (Men who took prophylactic aspirin therapy had a 56% lower risk of developing an MI during the follow-up period.) The baseline CRP level was an independent predictor of such thrombotic risk.

Limitation of C-reactive protein as a marker

Although CRP may be a useful marker, its measurement within the normal range is dependent on ultrasensitive enzyme immunoassays, and there is often large intra-patient variablity with routine laboratory measurements.[70] Also, CRP's acute phase response is a non-specific phenomenon induced by almost all forms of tissue damage and inflammation, and is certainly not limited to atherosclerosis.

Leucocyte integrins

The term 'integrins' was coined by Hynes in 1987[71] for a group of integral membrane glycoprotein receptors thought to 'integrate' the cytoskeleton of one cell with either that of another cell or with the extracellular matrix. The integrins comprise a superfamily of heterodimer transmembrane proteins composed of non-covalently associated α- and β-subunits.[72]

CD11b and CD11c

The leucocyte integrins, CD11b and CD11c, are glycoproteins expressed mainly on monocytes and tissue macrophages. CD11b and CD11c have receptors for binding immobilised fibrinogen and intercellular adhesion molecule-1 [ICAM-1]; the latter is involved in monocyte adhesion, recruitment and migration in areas of inflammation and atherogenesis.[73]

CD11b molecules (which appear to be functionally more important than CD11c) are induced by inflammation.[74] CD11b is stored in secretory granules in monocytes (as well as neutrophils) and can be rapidly mobilised to the cell surface after cell activation, such that the number of binding sites per cell may then increase four- to fivefold.[75] Enhanced monocyte expression of CD11b facilitates the adhesion of these cells to endothelium, extracellular matrix and iC3b-a crucial step in the pathogenesis of vascular injury.[76] Both CD11b and CD11c have also been shown to participate in thrombus formation. The binding of these molecules to immobilised fibrinogen induces the transcription of the tissue factor gene in monocytes, resulting in enhanced surface expression of tissue factor, and so increases the procoagulant activity of these cells.[77] Monocytes can also initiate coagulation and generate thrombin via another pathway: Altieri and Edgington showed that these cells can directly activate factor X to Xa after binding this zymogen to CD11b.[78]

Mazzone *et al.* measured CD11b expression on granulocytes and monocytes obtained from the coronary sinus and aorta in the course of cardiac catheterisation of patients with stable angina, unstable angina or non-cardiac chest pain.[79] Expression of CD11b was greater in patients with unstable angina than in the other groups, a finding consistent with the presence of inflammation within the coronary arteries of these patients. In addition, Mickelson *et al.* demonstrated that in patients who had undergone coronary angioplasty procedures, there was evidence of increased leucocyte activation, as indicated by the enhanced CD11b surface expression on monocytes and neutrophils.[80] The increased cell activation in such patients correlated with a higher risk of experiencing an adverse cardiac event.

Tissue factor

Tissue factor, a integral membrane glycoprotein comprising 263 amino acids, is expressed on the surface of monocytes (as well as on smooth muscle and endothelial cells) after these cells are stimulated by endotoxin[81] or by any of a variety of immunological[82,83] and inflammatory stimuli.[84] Tissue factor serves as a cofactor for the activation of factor VII to factor VIIa, so initiating intrinsic and extrinsic pathways of the coagulation system.[85]

Extensive *in vitro* studies have shown that inflammatory agents and mediators of the inflammatory response induce tissue factor expression in both monocytes and endothelial cells.[86,87] Enhanced tissue factor-induced procoagulant activity of monocytes has been described in several medical disorders associated with hypercoagulability, including sepsis, autoimmune disorders and cancer.[83,88–90] Furthermore, a comparable increase in procoagulant activity has also been observed in patients with unstable angina.[91]

In vitro infection of endothelial cells with either herpes simplex virus[92] or cytomegalovirus (CMV)[93] has been shown to increase procoagulant activity via tissue factor upregulation. Similarly, *C. pneumoniae*-infected arterial endothelial cells displayed enhanced tissue factor procoagulant activity *in vitro*.[94] Using a whole blood method assay, Leatham *et al.* found elevated tissue factor expression on the monocytes of patients with acute and chronic CHD.[95] These workers speculated that the increased tissue factor activity could be a result of chronic *C. pneumoniae* infection (see Figure 2).

Figure 2: Tissue factor-mediated activation of the coagulation system

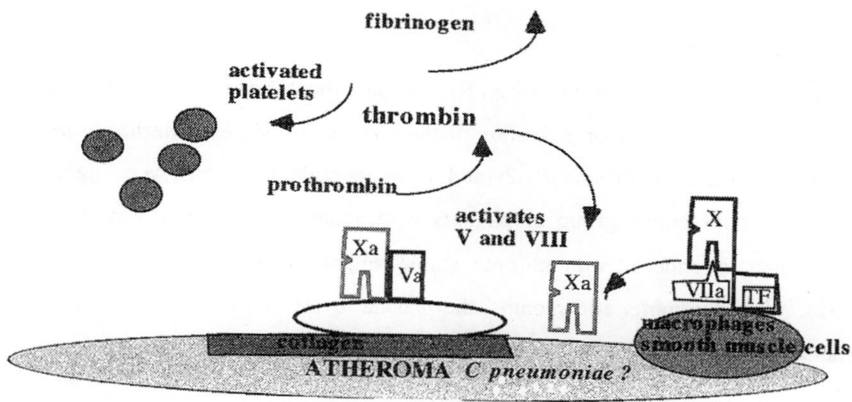

Expression of tissue factor on macrophages and monocytes leading to the activation of both the intrinsic and extrinsic coagulation pathways in atherothrombosis, a process possibly initiated by a local chronic infection with *C. pneumoniae*.

Fibrinogen

The Northwick Park Heart Study[96] and several prospective studies[97–100] have provided evidence for an independent relationship between raised plasma fibrinogen levels and increased incidence of CHD and stroke. In the PROspective CArdiovascular Munster (PROCAM) study,[100] for example, the higher a patient's baseline fibrinogen level, the greater the risk of a coronary event occurring during a subsequent 6-year follow-up period.

Mechanisms by which fibrinogen could promote CHD include: direct effect on atherogenesis, alteration of whole blood and plasma viscosity, and enhancing platelet aggregability and fibrin deposition. In addition, elevated fibrinogen levels in patients with CHD may reflect the underlying inflammatory component of atherosclerosis.

Thrombin fragments

The activation peptide of prothrombin, F1.2, is an indicator of thrombin generation and a direct marker of degree of activation of the coagulation system. Merlini *et al.* found that concentrations of plasma F1.2 (and fibrinopeptide A) levels were significantly higher in a consecutive group of patients with acute MI (n=32) or unstable angina (n=81) than in patients with chronic stable angina (n=37) or in healthy controls (n=32).[101] Furthermore, at 6 months, the plasma levels of F1.2 remained persistently higher in the group with acute coronary syndromes.

Neopterin

Investigation of the cytokine cascade of the human immune system *in vivo* (e.g. in the context of atherogenesis) is complicated by the fact that most of these mediators are biologically labile, and, after release, bind to target cells or disappear rapidly from the circulation.[102] An alternative indirect approach for monitoring cytokine activity is to quantify biochemical changes induced by these mediators. For instance, the concentration of neopterin, a monocyte/macrophage-derived, biologically stable product induced by interferon-γ, is a non-specific marker of the activity of the cell-mediated immune system.[103] Accordingly, serum levels of neopterin tend to be raised in patients with viral, parasitic or intracellular bacterial infections,[104] tend to correlate with the severity of the clinical condition, and so fall following eradication of such infection.[105] Neopterin levels also tend to be elevated in inflammatory and autoimmune disorders[106] and in malignancy (particularly that involving haematological cells).[107] Raised serum neopterin levels have also been found in acute MI,[108] acute coronary syndromes,[109] cardiomyopathies[110] and peripheral atherosclerosis.[111] Such elevations may reflect the immune activation now known to accompany these cardiac conditions.

Summary

Current evidence indicates that atherosclerosis is essentially the result of an exaggerated inflammatory response to injury of the endothelial cells in the arterial wall. The formation of atherosclerotic plaques can begin at an early age, especially in people exposed to atherogenic risk factors. Risk of plaque rupture – leading to acute thrombosis – appears to depend primarily on factors such as plaque geometry and compostion (rather than plaque volume/size), with inflammation playing a major destabilising role. Although risk factors such as cholesterol, smoking and diabetes mellitus may help to initiate atherogenesis, several rheological, haemostatic and inflammatory mediators appear more closely associated with disease progression, plaque 'activity', thrombosis and acute coronary events.

Whether infective agents provide a plausible link between atherogenesis, inflammation and progression of CHD is the focus of the next chapter.

References

1. Boaz A, Rayner M. *Coronary Heart Disease Statistics*, British Heart Foundation/Coronary Prevention Group. Statistics Database; 1995.
2. Hennekens CH. Increasing burden of cardiovascular disease: current knowledge and future directions for research on risk factors. *Circulation* 1998; **97**: 1095–102.
3. *Statistical Abstract of the United States: 1995*. US Department of Commerce, Washington, DC, USA; 1995.
4. Tunstall-Pedoe H, Kuulasmaa K, Amouyel P *et al.* Myocardial infarction and coronary deaths in the WHO MONICA project. Registration procedures, event rates and case-fatality rates in 38 populations from 21 countries in 4 continents. *Circulation* 1994; **90**: 583–612.
5. Buja LM. Does atherosclerosis have an infectious eitology? *Circulation* 1996; **94**: 872–3.
6. Nieminen MS, Mattila K, Valtonen V. Infection and inflammation as risk factors for myocardial infarction. *Eur Heart J* 1993; **14**(Suppl K): 12–6.
7. Sumpter MT, Dunn MI. Is coronary artery disease an infectious disease? *Chest* 1997; **112**: 302–3.
8. Keys A. Seven countries – a multivariate analysis of death and coronary heart disease. Harvard University Press, Boston, USA; 1980.
9. Criqui MH, Ringel BL. Does diet or alcohol explain the French paradox? *Lancet* 1994; **344**: 1719–23.
10. Reddy KS. Coronary heart disease in different racial groups. In: *Advanced Issues in Prevention and Treatment of Atherosclerosis* (Yusuf S, Wilhelmsen L, eds). Euromed Communications Ltd Publishers, Surrey, UK, 1995; pp. 47–60.
11. Barker DJ. Fetal origins of coronary heart disease. *BMJ* 1995; **311**: 171–4.
12. Reaven GM. Banting Lecture 1988: Role of insulin resistance in human disease. *Diabetes* 1998; **37**: 35–41.
13. Malinow MR. Homocysteine and arterial occlusive diseases. *J Intern Med* 1994; **236**: 603–17.
14. Stamler JS, Slivka A. Biological chemistry of thiols in the vasculature and in vascular-related disease. *Nutr Rev* 1996; **54**: 1–30.
15. Nygard O, Nordrehaug JE, Refsum H *et al.* Plasma homocysteine levels and mortality in patients with coronary artery disease. *N Engl J Med* 1997; **337**: 230–6.
16. Harrap SB, Watt GCM. Genetics and risk of coronary heart disease. *Med J Aust* 1992; **156**: 594–6.
17. Wood D, De Backer G, Faergeman O *et al.* Prevention of coronary heart disease in clinical practice: Recommendations of the second joint task force of European and other Societies on coronary prevention. *Eur Heart J* 1998; **19**: 1434–503.
18. Gupta S, Camm AJ. *Chlamydia pneumoniae* and coronary heart disease: coincidence, association or causation? *BMJ* 1997; **314**: 1778–9.
19. Falk E, Shah PK, Fuster V. Coronary plaque disruption. *Circulation* 1995; **92**: 657–71.
20. Ambrose JA, Tannenbaum MA, Alexopoulos D *et al.* Angiographic progression of coronary artery disease and the development of myocardial infarction. *J Am Coll Cardiol* 1988; **12**: 56–62.
21. Rokitansky C von. *A Manual of Pathological Anatomy*, Day GE (translator). Vol. 4, The Sydenham Society, London, UK; 1852.
22. Virchow R. Phloge und Thrombose in Gefassystem, gesammelte Bahandlungen zur wissenschaftlichen Medicin. Meidinger Sohn and Co. Frankfurt-am-Main, Germany, 1856; p. 458.
23. Duguid JB. Thrombosis as a factor in the pathogenesis of coronary atherosclerosis. *J Pathol Bacteriol* 1946; **58**: 207.
24. Benditt EP, Benditt JM. Evidence for a monoclonal origin of human atherosclerotic plaques. *Proc Natl Acad Sci USA* 1993; **70**: 1753–6.

25. Ross R, Glomset J. Atherosclerosis and the arterial smooth muscle cell. Proliferation of smooth muscle is a key event in the genesis of the lesions of atherosclerosis. *Science* 1973; **180**: 1332–9.
26. Ross R. The pathogenesis of atherosclerosis: A perspective for the 1990s. *Nature* 1993; **362**: 801–9.
27. Vogel RA. Coronary risk factors, endothelial function and atherosclerosis: A review. *Clin Cardiol* 1997; **20**: 426–32.
28. Mora R, Lupu F, Simionescu N. Prelesional events in atherogenesis. Colonisation of apolipoprotein B, unesterised cholesterol and extracellular phospholipid liposomes in the aorta of hyperlipidemic rabbit. *Atherosclerosis* 1987; **67**: 143–54.
29. Munro JM, Cotran RS. The pathogenesis of atherosclerosis: Atherogenesis and inflammation. *Lab Invest* 1988; **58**: 249–61.
30. Nilsson J. Growth factors and the pathogenesis of atherosclerosis. *Atherosclerosis* 1986; **62**: 185–99.
31. Steinberg D, Parathasarthy S, Carew TE, Khoo JC, Witztum JL. Beyond cholesterol. Modifications of LDL that increase its atherogenicity. *N Engl J Med* 1989; **320**: 915–24.
32. Faggiotto A, Ross R, Harker L. Studies of hypercholesterolaemia in the non-human primate. I. Changes that lead to fatty streak formation. *Arteriosclerosis* 1984; **4**: 323–40.
33. Rosenfeld ME, Tsukada T, Gown AM, Ross R. Fatty streak initiation in Wantanabe Heritable Hyperlipemic and comparably hypercholesterolemic fat-fed rabbits *Arteriosclerosis* 1987; **7**: 9–23.
34. Masuda J, Ross R. Atherogenesis during low level hypercholesterolaemia in the non-human primate. I. Fatty streak formation. *Arteriosclerosis* 1990; **10**: 164–77.
35. Berenson GS, Wattingney WA, Tracey RE *et al.* Atherosclerosis of the aorta and coronary arteries and cardiovascular risk factors in persons aged 6 to 30 years and studied at necropsy (The Bogalusa Heart Study). *Am J Cardiol* 1992; **70**: 851–8.
36. Brown MS, Goldstein JL. Lipoprotein metabolism in the macrophage: implications for cholesterol deposition in atherosclerosis. *Ann Rev Biochem* 1983; **52**: 223–61.
37. Thomas WA, Lee KT, Kim DN. Cell population kinetics in atherogenesis. Cell births and losses in intimal cell mass-derived lesions in the abdominal aorta of swine. *Ann N Y Acad Sci* 1985; **454**: 305–15.
38. Azar RR, Waters DD. The inflammatory etiology of unstable angina. *Am Heart J* 1996; **132**: 1101–6.
39. Battegay EJ, Raines EW, Seifert RA, Bowen-Pope DF, Ross R. TGF-beta induces bimodal proliferation of connective tissue cells via complex control of an autocrine PDGF loop. *Cell* 1990; **63**: 515–24.
40. Ross R, Raines EW, Bowen-Pope DF. The biology of platelet-derived growth factor. *Cell* 1986; **46**: 155–69.
41. Faruqi RM, DiCorleto PE. Mechanisms of monocyte recruitment and accumulation. *Br Heart J* 1993; **69** (Suppl 1): S19–S29.
42. Valente AJ, Rozek MM, Sprague EA, Schwartz CJ. Mechanisms in intimal monocyte–macrophage recruitment. *Circulation* 1992; **86** (Suppl III): 20–5.
43. O'Brien KD, Chait A. The biology of the artery wall in atherogenesis. *Med Clin North Am* 1994; **78**: 41–67.
44. Munro JM. Endothelial–leukocyte adhesive interations in inflammatory diseases. *Eur Heart J* 1993; **14** (Suppl K): S72–7.
45. Hansson GK. Immune and inflammatory mechanisms in the development of atherosclerosis. *Br Heart J* 1993; **69** (Suppl 1): S38–S42.
46. Hansson GK, Jonasson L, Seifert PS, Stemme S. Immune mechanisms in atheroscelerosis. *Arteriosclerosis* 1989; **9**: 567–78.
47. Emeson EE, Robertson AL Jr. T-lymphocytes in aortic and coronary intimas. Their potential role in atherogenesis. *Am J Pathol* 1988; **130**: 369–76.

48. Clinton SK, Libby P. Cytokines and growth factors in atherogenesis. *Arch Pathol Lab Med* 1992; **116**: 1292–300.
49. Fuster V, Badimon L, Badimon JJ, Chesebro JH. The pathogenesis of coronary artery disease and the acute coronary syndromes. *N Engl J Med* 1992; **326**: 310–8.
50. Friedman GD, Klatsky AL, Siegelaub AB. The leukocyte count as a predictor of myocardial infarction. *N Engl J Med* 1974; **290**: 1275–8.
51. Zalokar JB, Richard JL, Claude JR. Leukocyte count, smoking and myocardial infarction. *N Engl J Med* 1981; **394**: 465–8.
52. Yarnell JW, Baker IA, Sweetnam PM *et al.* Fibrinogen, viscosity, and white blood cell count are major risk factors for ischemic heart disease. The Caerphilly and Speedwell collaborative heart disease studies. *Circulation* 1991; **83**: 836–44.
53. Phillips AN, Neaton JD, Cook DG, Grimm RH, Shaper AG. Leukocyte count and risk of major coronary heart disease events. *Am J Epidemiol* 1992; **136**: 59–70.
54. Grimm RH, Neaton JD, Ludwig W *et al.* Prognostic importance of the white blood cell count for coronary, cancer, and all-cause mortality. *JAMA* 1985; **254**: 1932–7.
55. Kawaguchi H, Mori T, Kawano T *et al.* Band neutrophil count and the presence and severity of coronary atherosclerosis. *Am Heart J* 1996; **132**: 9–12.
56. Ernst E, Hammerschmidt DE, Bagge U, Matrai A, Dormandy JA. Leukocytes and the risk of ischaemic disease. *JAMA* 1987; **257**: 2318–24.
57. Craddock PR, Hammerschmidt DE, White JG, Dalmosso AP, Jacob HS. Complement (C5a)-induced granulocyte aggregation *in vitro*: A possible mechanism of complement-mediated leukostasis amd leukopenia. *J Clin Invest* 1977; **60**: 260–4.
58. Weissman G, Smolen JE, Korchak HM. Release of inflammatory mediators from stimulated neutrophils. *N Engl J Med* 1980; **303**: 27–34.
59. Sacks T, Moldow CF, Craddock PR, Bowers TK, Jacob HS. Oxygen radical-mediated endothelial cell damage by complement-stimulated granulocytes: an *in vitro* model of immune vascular damage. *J Clin Invest* 1978; **61**: 1161–7.
60. Prentice RL, Szatrowski TP, Fujikura T *et al.* Leukocyte counts and coronary heart disease in a Japanese cohort. *Am J Epidemiol* 1982; **116**: 496–509.
61. Olivares R, Ducimetiere P, Claude JR. Monocyte count: a risk factor for coronary heart disease. *Am J Epidemiol* 1993; **137**: 49–53.
62. Pepys MB, Baltz ML. Acute phase proteins with special reference to C-reactive protein and related proteins (pentaxins) and serum amyloid A protein. *Adv Immunol* 1983; **34**: 141–212.
63. Pepys MB. The acute phase response and C-reactive protein. In: *Oxford Textbook of Medicine*, 3rd edn (Weatherall DJ, Ledingham JGG, Warrell DA, eds). Oxford University Press, Oxford, UK, 1995; pp. 1527–33.
64. Heinrich J, Schulte H, Schonfeld R, Kohler E, Assmann G. Association of variables of coagulation, fibrinolysis and acute-phase with atherosclerosis in coronary and peripheral arteries and those arteries supplying the brain. *Thromb Haemost* 1995; **73**: 374–9.
65. Liuzzo G, Biasucci LM, Gallimore JR *et al.* The prognostic value of C-reactive and serum amyloid A protein in severe unstable angina. *N Engl J Med* 1994; **331**: 417–24.
66. Haverkate F, Thompson SG, Pyke SD, Gallimore JR, Papys MB. Production of C-reactive protein and risk of coronary events on stable and unstable angina. *Lancet* 1997; **349**: 462–6.
67. Mendall MA, Patel P, Ballam L *et al.* C reactive protein and its relation to cardiovascular risk factors: a population based cross sectional study. *BMJ* 1996; **312**: 1061–5.
68. Patel P, Mendall MA, Carrington D *et al.* Association of *Helicobacter pylori* and *Chlamydia pneumoniae* infections with coronary heart disease and cardiovascular risk factors *BMJ* 1995; **311**: 711–4.
69. Ridker PM, Cushman M, Stampfer MJ, Tracy RP, Hennekens CH. Inflammation, aspirin and the risk of cardiovascular disease in apparently healthy men. *N Engl J Med* 1997; **336**: 973–9.

70. Sewell WA, Bird AG, Marshall SE, Chapel HM. Relation of C reactive protein to cardiovascular risk factors: Assays would have to be developed to measure C reactive protein. *BMJ* 1996; **313**: 428 [letter].
71. Hynes RO. Integrins: a family of cell surface receptors. *Cell* 1987; **48**: 549–54.
72. Sanchez-Madrid F, Nagy JA, Robbins E, Simon P, Springer TA. A human leukocyte differentiation antigen family with distinct alpha-subunits and a common beta subunit: The lymphocyte function-associated (LFA-1), the C3bi complement receptor (OKM1/mac-1) and the p150,95 molecule. *J Exp Med* 1983; **158**: 1785–803.
73. Jang Y, Lincoff AM, Plow EF, Topol EJ. Cell adhesion molecules in coronary artery disease. *J Am Coll Cardiol* 1994; **24**: 1591–601.
74. Smith CW, Rothlein R, Hughes BJ *et al.* Recognition of an endothelial determinant for CD18-dependent human neutrophil adherence and transendothelial migration. *J Clin Invest* 1988; **82**: 1746–56.
75. Hughes BJ, Hollers CJ, Crockett-Torabi E *et al.* Recruitment of CD11b/CD18 to neutrophil surface and adherence-dependent cell locomotion. *J Clin Invest* 1992; **90**: 1687–96.
76. Tonnesen MG, Smedly LA, Henson PM. Neutrophil-endothelial cell interactions. *J Clin Invest* 1984; **74**: 1581–92.
77. Fan ST, Edgington TS. Coupling of the adhesive receptor CD11b/CD18 to functional enhancement of effector macrophage tissue factor response. *J Clin Invest* 1991; **87**: 50–7.
78. Altieri DC, Edgington TS. The saturable high affinity association of factor X to ADP-stimulated monocytes defines a novel function of the Mac-1 receptor. *J Biol Chem* 1991; **263**: 7007–15.
79. Mazzone A, De Servi S, Ricevuti G *et al.* Increased expression of neutrophil and monocyte adhesion molecules in unstable coronary artery disease. *Circulation* 1993; **88**: 358–63.
80. Michelson JK, Lakkis NM, Villarreal-Levy G, Hughes BJ, Smith CW. Leukocyte activation with platelet adhesion after coronary angioplasty: A mechanism for recurrent disease. *J Am Coll Cardiol* 1996; **28**: 345–53.
81. Rivers RP, Hathaway WE, Weston WL. The endotoxin-induced coagulant activity of human monocytes. *Br J Haematol* 1975; **30**: 311–6.
82. Drake TA, Hannani K, Fei H, Lavi S, Berliner JA. Minimally oxidized low-density lipoprotein induces tissue factor expression in cultured human endothelial cells. *Am J Pathol* 1991; **138**: 601–7.
83. Lyberg T, Prydz H, Baklien K, Hoyeraal HM. Effects of immune complex-containing sera from patients with rheumatic diseases on thromboplastin activity of monocytes. *Thromb Res* 1982; **25**: 193–202.
84. Kornberg A, Catane R, Peller S, Kaufman S, Fridkin M. Tuftsin induces tissue factor-like activity in human mononuclear cells and in monocytic cell lines. *Blood* 1990; **76**: 814–9.
85. Nemerson Y. Tissue factor and hemostasis. *Blood* 1988; **71**: 1–8.
86. Brozna JP. Cellular regulation of tissue factor. *Blood Coag* 1990; **1**: 415–26.
87. Bevilacqua MP, Gimbrone MA Jr. Inducible endothelial functions in inflammation and coagulation. *Sem Thromb Haemost* 1987; **13**: 425–33.
88. Rivers RP, Cattermole HE, Wright I. The expression of surface tissue factor apoprotein by blood monocytes in the course of infections in early infancy. *Pediatr Res* 1992; **31**: 567–73.
89. Osterud B, Flaegstad T. Increased tissue thromboplastin activity in monocytes of patients with meningococcal infection: related to an unfavourable prognosis. *Thromb Haemost* 1983; **49**: 5–7.
90. Lorenzet R, Peri G, Locati D *et al.* Generation of procoagulant activity by mononuclear phagocytes: a possible mechanism contributing to blood clotting activation within malignant tissues. *Blood* 1983; **62**: 271–3.
91. Serneri GG, Abbate R, Gori AM *et al.* Transient intermittent lymphocyte activation is responsible for the instability of unstable angina. *Circulation* 1992; **86**: 790–7.

92. Key NS, Vercellotti GM, Winkelmann JC *et al.* Infection of vascular endothelial cells with herpes simplex virus enhances tissue factor activity and reduces thrombomodulin expression. *Proc Natl Acad Sci USA* 1990; **87**: 7095–9.
93. Dam-Mieras Van DC, Muller AD, Hinsbergh VW *et al.* The procoagulant response of cytomegalovirus infected endothelial cells. *Thromb Haemost* 1992; **68**: 364–70.
94. Fryer RH, Schwobe EP, Woods ML, Rodgers GM. *Chlamydia* species infect human vascular endothelial cells and induce procoagulant activity. *J Invest Med* 1997; **45**: 168–74.
95. Leatham EW, Bath PM, Tooze JA, Camm AJ. Increased monocyte tissue factor expression in coronary disease. *Br Heart J* 1995; **73**: 10–3.
96. Meade TW, Fellows S, Brozovic M *et al.* Haemostatic function and ischaemic heart disease: principal results of the Northwick Park Heart Study. *Lancet* 1986; **2**: 533–72.
97. Wilhelmsen L, Svardsudd K, Korsan-Bengsten K *et al.* Fibrinogen as a risk factor for stroke and myocardial infarction. *N Engl J Med* 1984; **311**: 501–5.
98. Thompson S, Kienast J, Pyke S, Heverkate F, Van de Loo J. Hemostatic factors and the risk of myocardial infarction and sudden death in patients with angina pectoris. *N Engl J Med* 1995; **332**: 635–41.
99. Kannel WB, Wolf PA, Castelli WP, D'Agostino RB. Fibrinogen and risk of cardiovascular disease. The Framingham Study. *JAMA* 1987; **258**: 1183–6.
100. Heinrich J, Balleisen L, Schulte H, Assmann G, Van de Loo J. Fibrinogen and factor VII in the prediction of coronary risk. Results from the PROCAM study in healthy men. *Arterioscler Thromb* 1994; **14**: 54–9.
101. Merlini PA, Bauer KA, Oltrona L *et al.* Persistent activation of coagulation mechanism in unstable angina and myocardial infarction. *Circulation* 1994; **90**: 61–8.
102. Engelberts I, Moller A, Schoen GJ, Van der Linden CJ, Burman WA. Evaluation of measurement of human TNF in plasma by ELISA. *Lymphokine Cytokine Res* 1991; **10**: 69–76.
103. Fuchs D, Weiss G, Wachter H. Neopterin, biochemistry and clinical use as a marker for cellular immune reactions. *Int Arch Allergy Immunol* 1993; **101**: 1–6.
104. Hausen A, Fuchs D, Reibnegger G *et al.* Neopterin in clinical use. *Pteridines* 1989; **1**: 3–10.
105. Carstens J, Andersen PL. Changes in serum neopterin and serum beta 2-microglobulin in subjects with lung infections. *Eur Respir J* 1994; **7**: 1233–8.
106. Schwedes U, Teuber J, Schmidt R, Usadel KH. Neopterin as a marker for the activity of antoimmune thyroid diseases. *Acta Endocrinol* 1986; **111**: 51–2.
107. Denz H, Grunewald K, Thaler J *et al.* Urinary neopterin as a prognostic marker in haematological neoplasias. *Pteridines* 1989; **1**: 167–70.
108. Melichar B, Gregor J, Solichova D *et al.* Increased urinary neopterin in acute myocardial infarction. *Clin Chem* 1994; **40**: 338–9.
109. Gupta S, Fredericks S, Schwartzman RA *et al.* Serum neopterin in acute coronary syndromes. *Lancet* 1997: **349**: 1252–3 [letter].
110. Samsonov M, Fuchs D, Reibnegger G *et al.* Patterns of serological markers for cellular immune activation in patients with dilated cardiomyopathy and chronic myocarditis. *Clin Chem* 1992; **38**: 678–80.
111. Tatzber F, Rabl H, Koriska K *et al.* Elevated serum neopterin levels in atherosclerosis. *Atherosclerosis* 1991; **89**: 203–8.

Chapter 2: Associations between infective microorganisms and atherosclerosis

Introduction

The idea that infection could be a causal factor in the pathogenesis of atherosclerosis is not new. Indeed, Sir William Osler and others first proposed such a mechanism as long ago as 1908.[1] Until recently, however, the suggestion had largely been dismissed. Fresh debate now focuses on whether or not common chronic infections contribute to the development and progression of atherosclerotic disease, not least because epidemiological variations in classical cardiovascular risk factors such as smoking, diabetes mellitus and hypercholesterolaemia do not account for the variations in the presence and severity of coronary heart disease (CHD) seen in the general population (see Chapter 1).[2–4] In addition, *in vitro* experiments, animal studies, pathological examinations and clinical observations provide supporting evidence for associations between infectious diseases and atherosclerosis.[5] At the same time, increasing understanding of inflammatory and haemostatic mediators and of the monocyte/macrophage system's role in atherogenesis have facilitated research into whether or not infections have a direct pathogenetic role in CHD. In essence, while an inflammatory basis to atherosclerosis and CHD is now generally acknowledged,[6] an aetiological role for chronic infections, through highly plausible, is by no means proven.

It is interesting to observe how an increasing number of chronic inflammatory conditions have been associated with infective aetiologies – although the weight of supporting evidence varies markedly from disease to disease (see Table 1).

Table 1: The potential association between chronic inflammatory diseases and infection

Disease	**Infective agent**
Peptic ulcers	*Helicobacter pylori*[7]
Rheumatoid arthritis	Herpesviruses[8]
Crohn's disease	*Mycobacterium paratuberculosis*[9]
Multiple sclerosis	Herpesviruses[10]
Sarcoidosis	*Mycobacterium*[11]

How might infections be involved?

The 'response-to-injury' hypothesis of atherosclerosis acknowledges that infection could trigger and aggravate endothelial damage.[12] However, there are also several other mechanisrns, by which infections might directly or indirectly initiate or perpetuate atherosclerosis or its complications (see Table 2). These include: microorganism-related damage of endothelial cells, stimulation of atherogenic inflammatory responses and faciliatation of thrombosis.

Endothelial cells might become directly infected. In accordance with this idea, human umbilical endothelial cell cultures are susceptible to *in vitro* infection with cytomegalovirus (CMV),[13] herpes simplex virus (HSV-1),[14] echovirus[15] and *Chlamydia pneumoniae*.[16] Endotoxin (secreted by bacteria), immune complexes or circulating lipid-endotoxin complexes may directly damage the endothelium. For instance, endotoxin triggers vascular damage in rabbit[17] and pig[18] models of atherosclerosis. Endotoxin also binds to lipoproteins in the circulation, some of which are then avidly taken up by macrophages. Subsequent activation of the macrophages (or of smooth muscle cells) may lead to production of cytokines, major histocompatibility complex (MHC) upregulation and synthesis of acute phase proteins, such as fibrinogen and C-reactive protein (CRP) – processes which could perpetuate an atherogenic inflammatory response.[19] Production of tissue necrosis factor-α and interleukin-1 may alter cholesterol metabolism[20] and induce further recruitment of inflammatory cells to atherosclerotic plaques. Infections may also directly affect cholesterol metabolism and lipid oxidation,[21] so leading to a more atherogenic lipid profile. Another possibility is that low-grade chronic infection may lead to a hypercoaguable state, via activation of monocytes with resulting increased tissue factor expression.[22] Infection of endothelial cells *in vivo* may increase thrombin generation on the cell surface, increase platelet accumulation or reduce prostacyclin secretion – effects which could increase the risk of local or distal thrombosis.[23]

Table 2: Mechanisms by which infections might contribute to atherogenesis

Mechanism
Direct endothelial cell damage
Lipoprotein disturbances
Monocyte activation and cytokine production
Increased synthesis of acute phase proteins
Enhanced activity of procoagulant mediators
Heat shock protein expression

Which infections?

Several infective agents have been suggested as having a role in CHD. These include: herpesviruses, *H. pylori*, bacterial causes of dental sepsis, viral respiratory infections and *C. pneumoniae*.

Herpesvirus infections

Evidence from animal models

A clear association between an infectious agent and arterial disease is seen with Marek's disease in chickens. Marek's disease virus is an avian herpesvirus that causes lymphoproliferative disease in chickens. Early observations indicated that chickens 'naturally infected' with this virus subsequently developed atherosclerotic lesions.[24] In 1978, Fabricant *et al.* demonstrated that inoculating chickens with Marek's disease virus led to aggressive deposition of lipids within the animals' coronary artery walls.[25] When the animals were concurrently fed a cholesterol-enriched diet, the vascular lesions changed, becoming fibro-proliferative and very similar in appearance to human atherosclerotic plaques.[26] The virus was demonstrable in the arterial walls using immunofluorescence techniques.[27] Furthermore, cultured chicken aortic smooth muscle cells infected with the virus contained higher amounts of cholesterol than non-infected cells.[28] Moreover, vaccination of chickens (with a turkey vaccine) before innoculation with the Marek's disease virus led to the formation of fewer than expected atherosclerotic lesions.[26]

In subsequent studies performed in Japanese quail, DNA sequences related to the Marek's disease virus genome (but no infectious virions) were found in the arterial plaque lesions of birds known to be genetically susceptible to atherosclerosis; birds relatively resistant to such disease lacked such DNA sequences.[29]

In a rat model, experimental deliberate balloon injury of the carotid artery in immunosuppressed animals followed by deliberate infection with CMV caused endothelial injury.[30] The virus was subsequently demonstrable within the neointima in the areas of endothelial denudation. Also, in a rat allograft model, early CMV infection after transplantation significantly enhanced the development of smooth muscle cell proliferation and allograft atherosclerosis.[31]

Cytomegalovirus in humans

The finding of herpesvirus-induced atherosclerosis in chickens prompted research investigating the possibility of an analogous role of such viruses in humans. The clearest candidate microorganism in this setting is CMV.

CMV infection is very common. In the USA, for example, the prevalence of antibodies to CMV is about 10–15% in the adolescent population, rising to 40–50% by age 35 years, and to over 60–70% in adults over 65 years of age. This age-related pattern resembles that of atherosclerosis.[32] As with other herpesviruses, infection with CMV, can become chronic and 'latent', although the site of such dormancy remains unclear. Periodic reactivation of the infection may occur, particularly in immunosuppressed patients.

Evidence of CMV in plaques

In 1983, Melnick *et al.* reported the presence of CMV antigens (though not infectious virus) in smooth muscle cells cultured from arterial specimens taken from patients who had undergone carotid endarterectomy.[33] Furthermore, in another study, virions morphologically resembling herpesviruses were detected (by direct electron microscope examination) in a small percentage (2.5%) of biopsy specimens from the ascending aorta of patients with atherosclerosis.[34]

By contrast, studies conducted using dot-blot and *in situ* hybridisation techniques found that CMV DNA positivity was lower in femoral and abdominal arterial samples from patients undergoing vascular surgery for arterial disease than in an autopsy-control group (44% versus 58%).[35] However, when a more sensitive detection technique polymerase chain reaction (PCR) was used, the proportion of positive samples in the vascular surgery group increased (to 90%), whereas the results in the control group were little changed (53% of samples positive).[36] Since both early and late regions of the CMV genome could be amplified in this study and other studies have demonstrated CMV DNA distributed widely in the vascular tree,[37] it has been suggested that the arterial wall may be a site of latent CMV infection. Such infection could lead to chronic changes that predispose to the development of atherosclerosis.[38] In keeping with these notions, herpesviruses genomic sequences and antigens have also been detected in coronary artery and thoracic aorta samples (obtained at autopsy from trauma victims aged 15–35 years) showing early atheromatous changes.[39]

Overall, in 16 published studies on CMV in vascular pathology samples there were only small differences in the proportion of atheromatous and non-atheromatous blood vessels positive for CMV (47% [283 of 607] versus 39% [154 of 398]), with a weighted odds ratio (OR) of 1.4 (95% confidence interval [CI] 1.0–1.9).[40] One possible explanation for this finding is that in some cases, CMV may initiate the atherosclerotic process but the organism subsequently becomes difficult to detect. Circumstantial evidence to support this idea comes from studies using the more sensitive PCR technique: overall CMV was detected in 57% (228 of 399) of atheromatous vessels compared with 36% (113 of 311) of control samples, yielding a weighted OR of about 2.5 (95% CI 1.6–3.5).[40]

Anti-cytomegalovirus antibodies and atherosclerotic disease

A significantly higher prevalence of serum anti-CMV antibodies and higher antibody titres have been observed among patients with vascular disease compared with controls without such disease but matched for age, ethnicity, hyperlipidaemia and socioeconomic background.[41] Similarly, in another study, high titres of anti-CMV antibodies were more prevalent among patients undergoing surgery for atherosclerotic disease (70%) than in matched control patients (43%).[42] A case–control study performed on a subset of the Atherosclerosis Risk in Communities (ARIC) study[43] indicated that those with carotid artery intimal thickening, on ultrasonographic examinations (a marker of 'preclinical' atherosclerosis), had significantly higher anti-CMV antibody titres than controls without such vessel thickening.[44] (There was no correlation between the presence or absence of intimal thickening and antibodies directed against HSV-1 or HSV-2 antigens.) This statistical association with CMV was not confounded by conventional CHD risk factors (hypercholesterolaemia, hypertension, diabetes mellitus). A subsequent prospective study in the ARIC cohort confirmed the relationship between raised anti-CMV antibody titre and increased risk of carotid wall thickening.[45] This contrasts with the negative findings of a further case–

control study.[46] Prior infection with CMV did not seem to be a significant risk factor for angiographically demonstrated CHD.

In a study conducted by Chiu *et al.*, CMV organisms were detected in over one-third of carotid atheroma samples, but the organism's presence showed no apparent correlation with serum levels of anti-CMV antibodies.[47]

Cytomegalovirus and post-angioplasty restenosis

The potential role for CMV in the restenosis of arteries that can follow coronary angioplasty has also been investigated.[48] In one study, histological examination of atheromatous tissue from restenotic areas revealed the presence of CMV DNA in 23 of 60 (38%) restenotic lesions examined. Smooth muscle cells from the restenosed lesion expressed CMV protein IE84 and contained high amounts of p53 (a tumour suppressor protein involved indirectly in DNA repair). Also, deliberate *in vitro* CMV infection of such smooth muscle cells led to enhanced p53 accumulation, which in turn had a temporal association with IE84 expression. These results support the findings of a prospective study conducted by Zhou *et al.*[49] These investigators found that patients with serological evidence of previous CMV infection had a high rate of restenosis after coronary angioplasty: 43% of those with anti-CMV IgG antibodies developed such restenosis compared with 8% of seronegative patients ($p<0.002$). The investigators suggested that, in certain patients, angioplasty-induced injury to the vessel wall may reactivate a latent CMV infection and enhance the smooth muscle cell proliferation (via IE84-mediated inhibition of p53 function) typically seen in restenotic lesions.

Other investigators were able to detect CMV DNA in only a small proportion of coronary endarterectomy specimens (two of 28 samples, 7%) taken during coronary artery bypass surgery.[50] Furthermore, Kol *et al.* were unable to demonstrate CMV messenger RNA in atherectomy specimens from 40 patients with CHD – evidence against the suggestion that locally active CMV infection plays a major pathogenetic role in atherogenesis.[51]

Cytomegalovirus in transplant vasculopathy

Stronger evidence that CMV plays a direct role in atherosclerosis comes from studies of the infection's association with the development of the accelerated allograft vasculopathy often seen in recipients of cardiac transplants.[52] This atherosclerotic process usually comprises diffuse smooth muscle proliferation, peri-vascular inflammation and collagen accumulation; classical atheromatous plaques are uncommon.[53]

Grattan reported on a series of 387 consecutive patients in Stanford, USA, who received heart transplants and had their CMV status checked (pre- and post-transplantation).[54] In all, 122 (32%) of the patients had serological evidence of CMV infection. Their clinical outcomes were compared with the remaining 265 transplant patients (the CMV-negative group). Transplant patients in the CMV-positive group developed atherosclerosis more often and earlier than seronegative patients. The actuarial mortality rate from atherosclerosis in the transplanted heart was 30% in this group compared to only 10% in the CMV-negative group ($p<0.05$). These observations have been confirmed by investigators in Minneapolis[55] and Baltimore.[56] These data are intriguing given that pathological studies have demonstrated CMV nucleic acids sequences (in addition to those of HSV virus and Epstein–Barr virus) in the coronary arteries of transplanted hearts.[57]

Overview

The suggestion that herpesviruses may have a role in atherogenesis is supported by *in vitro* studies. Infection of endothelial cells by herpesviruses results in a reduction in thrombomodulin expression and an increase in tissue factor activity,[58] changes which contribute to thrombosis in an atherosclerotic lesion. Furthermore, HSV-infected endothelial cells express the adhesion molecule GMP140 on their surface.[59] This molecule may in turn trigger adherence of leucocytes to endothelium, a feature of early atherosclerosis.

Although CMV is often detectable in human arterial tissue, there is no consistent association between CMV infection and atherosclerotic lesions in typical CHD patients. The finding of CMV antigens and nucleic acid sequences in arterial smooth muscle cells suggests that CMV infection of the arterial wall may be a common occurrence in patients with atherosclerosis. Although such findings form the basis of proposed pathogenetic mechanisms, by themselves they do not, of course, confirm a role for CMV in atherogenesis. Furthermore, since many individuals in the general population have antibody titres consistent with previous CMV infection (and, conversely, many patients with documented arterial diseases do not have elevated anti-CMV antibody titres), seroepidemiological data can hint at, but not prove, a causal relationship between CMV and atherosclerosis.[57]

A recent meta-analysis of the epidemiological associations between CMV and CHD identified several studies reporting odds ratios of 2 or higher (see Figure 3).[40] However, many of the studies considered involved small sample sizes, inadequate adjustments for known confounders and exploratory statistical analyses. In addition, fewer than 400 of the 1600 cases in these studies were defined as 'native' coronary atherosclerosis, with the majority involving cases of coronary artery restenosis, development of accelerated transplant atherosclerosis after transplantation or disease in arteries other than coronary arteries. There is much more evidence of a link between CMV infection and the development of accelerated transplant atherosclerosis,[54] (although not all studies support such an association[60]).

Figure 3: Epidemiological studies of CMV seropositivity and atherosclerotic disease

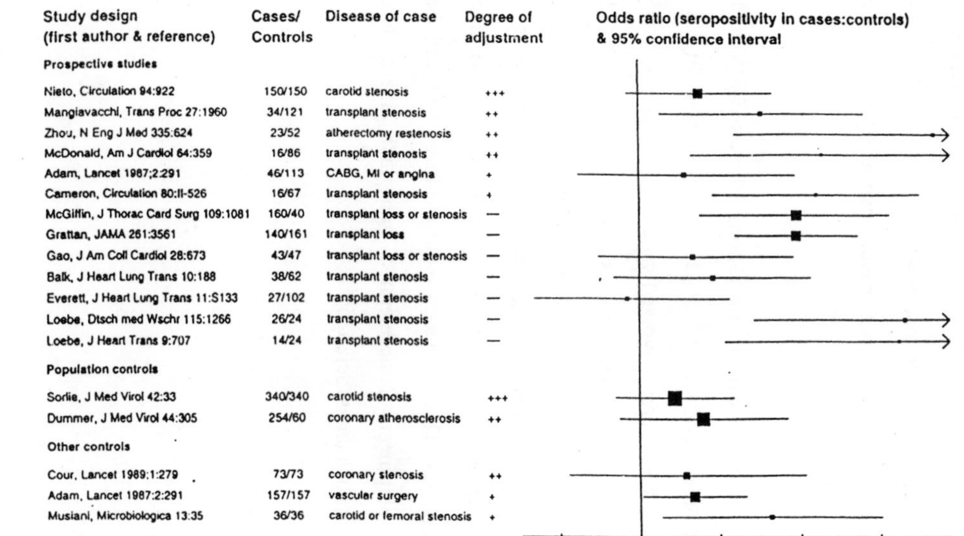

Degree of adjustment indicates which confounding variables were controlled for: + = age and gender alone; ++ = these and some vascular risk factors; +++ = these and markers of adult socioeconomic status; ++++ = these and markers of childhood socioeconomic status; CABG = coronary-artery bypass graft. Black squares indicate the OR, with the square size proportional to the number of cases, and horizontal lines represent 95% CI. (Adapted from Danesh J, Collins R, Peto R. Chronic infections and coronary heart disease: is there a link? *Lancet* 1997; **350**: 430–6, with permission.)

The biological properties of CMV are consistent with a pathogenetic involvement at different stages of atherogenesis, and many of these properties are shared by other herpesviruses. However, further investigation is required before these viruses can be said to have a role in human atherogenesis.

Helicobacter pylori

Helicobacter pylori is a bacterial infection, typically acquired in childhood, that colonises the stomach and causes peptic ulcer disease and type B gastritis.[61] Interest in a possible association between *H. pylori* and CHD originated from earlier observations of associations between peptic ulceration and CHD.[62]

Anti-*Helicobacter pylori* antibodies and CHD

In a case–control study conducted in London, UK, anti-*H. pylori* seropositivity correlated significantly with angiographically diagnosed CHD:[63] 66 of 111 (59%) males with CHD were seropositive for *H. pylori* compared with 29 of 74 (39%) controls (odds ratio 2.28; $p<0.007$). The same investigators went on to show that seropositivity to *H. pylori* was associated with serum cardiovascular risk markers, such as elevated leucocyte count, factor VIIa, C-reactive protein (CRP) and fibrinogen levels.[64] They postulated that the association between the organism and markers of cell activation and inflammation suggested mechanisms by which common infections could contribute to atherogenesis. In an alternative hypothesis, Birnie *et al.* proposed that an auto-immune process may explain the association between *H. pylori* and CHD.[65] They correlated the presence of both anti-heat shock protein 65 antibodies and that of anti-*H. pylori* antibodies with angiographically detected CHD. Furthermore, in a double-blind, placebo-controlled study, successful eradication of *H. pylori* led to a significant fall in anti-heat shock protein 65 antibody titres in the treated group.

Helicobacter pylori and CHD: confounding factors

Two studies have failed to show a relationship between coagulation and inflammatory markers and *H. pylori* infection.[66,67] Furthermore, larger studies using prospective methodologies and better-defined control subjects have been unable to demonstrate any independent association between this infection and CHD (see Figure 4).[68,69] These studies also suggested that lower socioeconomic status is a major confounding variable in any apparent relationship between *H. pylori* infection and atherosclerotic disease. Two prospective studies have attempted to establish whether there is a relationship between *H. pylori* and all-cause mortality risk. Strandberg *et al.*[70] investigated an elderly population of men and women (aged 75–85 years) over a 5-year period, while Strachan *et al.*[71] followed up middle-aged men for a period of 13.5 years. Both studies documented only weak associations between *H. pylori* seropositivity and mortality rates. These associations became statistically insignificant after adjustment of multiple covariates. On the basis of population prevalence data from developed nations, other observers have even suggested that there may be a negative association between seropositivity to *H. pylori* and deaths from CHD.[72]

A meta-analysis of 18 epidemiological studies, involving a total of over 10,000 patients, found no correlations between evidence of *H. pylori* infection and blood pressure, leucocyte count, or serum concentrations of total cholesterol, fibrinogen, triglycerides or C-reactive protein.[73] It has been suggested that the earlier claims of correlations between *H. pylori* seropositivity and certain vascular risk factors were largely, or wholly, due to chance or preferential publication of positive results.

Currently, there is no evidence to suggest that *H. pylori* is involved directly in the pathogenesis of atherosclerotic plaques. For example, one pathological study found no evidence of the organism in aortic plaque tissue analysed by PCR following removal from 51 patients undergoing abdominal aortic aneurysm surgery.[74] This was despite the fact that 92% of the patients had anti-*H. pylori* antibodies.

Figure 4: Epidemiological studies of *H. pylori* seropositivity and atherosclerotic disease

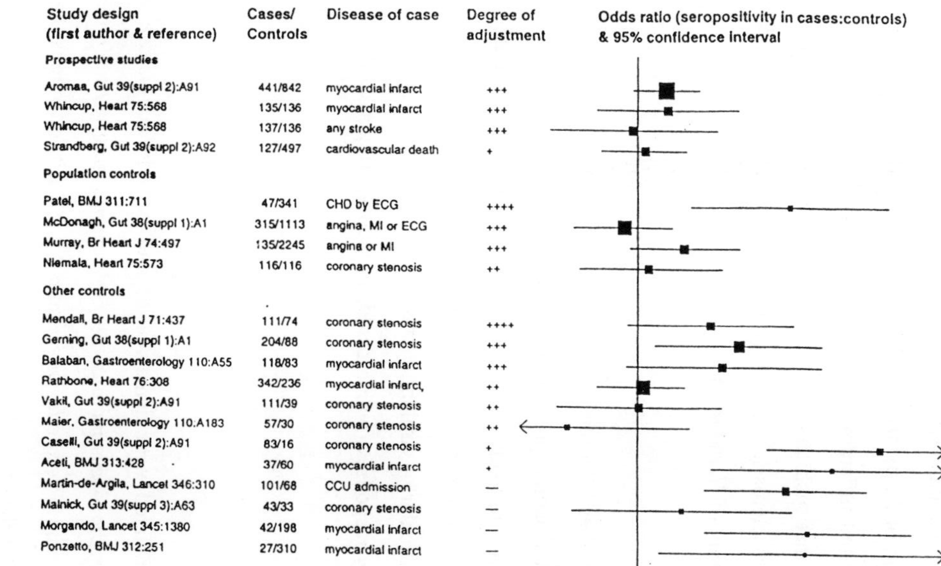

CCU = coronary care unit; ECG = electrocardiograph; MI = myocardial infarct. Other abbreviations and definitions as in Figure 3, page 32. (Adapted from Danesh J, Collins R, Peto R. Chronic infections and coronary heart disease: is there a link? *Lancet* 1997; **350:** 430–6, with permission.)

Virulent strains of *H. pylori* and CHD

A retrospective case–control study suggests that a particularly virulent form of *H. pylori*, the Cag-A (Cytotoxin-associated gene A) strain may be more clearly linked with CHD.[75] In this study, Pasceri *et al.* identified a significantly higher prevalence of the Cag-A positive strain of *H. pylori* in 88 patients with angiographically diagnosed CHD, than in 88 age- and sex-matched controls without CHD (43% versus 17%; $p<0.001$). It is worth noting that case subjects in this study were of lower socio-economic status than controls: this factor may have been acting as a major confounder in the apparent association of *H. pylori* and CHD. Given that the Cag-A strain may be associated with an increased inflammatory response (at least, in the setting of peptic ulceration), it is feasible that such an effect might, in the long term, have a bearing on the development of atherosclerosis.[6] Larger prospective studies are needed to clarify the role (if any) of this strain of *H. pylori* in CHD.

Overview

The early case–control studies[63] observing an association between *H. pylori* and CHD have been superseded by larger prospective investigations.[68,69] The latter studies indicate that the organism is unlikely to have a major independent role in atherogenesis or development of CHD. Whether or not a sub-group of seropositive subjects (say, those infected with particularly virulent strains of *H. pylori*[75]) mount abnormal immune or inflammatory responses (which could, in theory, trigger cardiac events) is not known.

Dental infections

Bacterial infections associated with dental caries and periodontal disease are most commonly caused by *Streptococcus mutans*, *Porphyromonas gingivalis*, *Actinobacillus actinomycetemcomitans* and *Prevotella intermedia*.[76,77] Such infections have been proposed as risk factors for the development of CHD.

Epidemiological data

An observational study by Mackenzie *et al.*[78] noted how a substantial number of patients with diabetes mellitus and atherosclerotic disease exhibited greater alveolar bone loss than that seen among healthy controls. Evidence from a later case–control study suggested that poor dental health could predispose to thromboembolic disorders: 40 patients presenting with acute cerbral infarction were noted to have a significantly higher prevalence of chronic dental infections than that in age- and sex-matched controls.[79]

The relationship between dental health and CHD was investigated by Mattila *et al.*[80] They scored the severity of dental infections according to a 'total dental index' (TDI), which was based on the number of carious teeth, extent of periodontal disease and number of periapical lesions. Overall, TDI was significantly higher in patients with recent myocardial infarction (MI) (n=100) compared with a matched series of controls (n=102). This association remained after adjustments were made for age, social class, smoking, serum lipid levels and diabetes mellitus. Similarly, in a large cross-sectional survey, around 1400 Finnish men who had lost over half of their teeth (an indirect marker of poor dental health) had a twofold increased risk of having a history of CHD compared with those who still had more than half of their own teeth.[81] This correlation was independent of age, height and educational status. Another study has suggested a positive (and independent) association between the extent of CHD (as scored on angiography) and the presence of dental sepsis.[82]

The authors of a meta-analysis commented on the increasing circumstantial evidence linking periodontal disease with CHD, especially in males aged 40–50 years.[83] It was, however, notable in this review that: nearly all the studies were performed exclusively in males; not all the studies specifically investigated periodontal disease (some used other measures such as number of teeth and radiological data); and not all the studies controlled adequately for established confounding atherogenic cardiovascular risk factors.

Possible mechanisms

There are several potential mechanisms by which dental sepsis might contribute to coronary atherogenesis. For example, the periodontal pocket typically contains between 10^7–10^8 bacteria, and the products of these bacteria (in particular the LPS and other endotoxins) will have ready access to the underlying vasculature of gingival connective tissue (and hence could undergo systemic spread).[83] In addition, Gram-negative bacteria may directly damage the endothelium. Indirect mechanisms may include a disturbance of the haemostatic system. Patients with poor dentition tend to have higher fibrinogen levels, leucocyte counts[84] and levels of other haemostatic markers including von Willebrand's factor antigen;[85] all of these factors might promote or contribute to atherothrombosis. Furthermore, some patients with periodontal disease may possess a particular monocyte phenotype associated with pro-inflammatory effects.[86]

Overview

Evidence of a clear relationship between dental health and CHD has emerged in observational studies. However, confirmatory prospective data are lacking, and the association between dental hygiene and CHD may simply reflect general health habits, rather than a causal relationship between dental sepsis and atherosclerosis. Whether dental disease simply mirrors other lifestyle factors more clearly associated with CHD, such as diet, exercise and smoking, needs further clarification.

Other infections associated with CHD

Acute respiratory infections

Seasonal variation occurs in the incidence of MI, with there being more hospital admissions during winter than summer months.[87] For example, in the Australian WHO MONICA trial registry, the incidence of fatal and non-fatal MI was 20–40% higher in the winter and spring months compared with the summer and autumn months. Similarly, it is estimated that there are about 20,000 additional deaths from cardiovascular disease each winter in England and Wales.[88] The influence of respiratory infections has been suggested as a cause of these variations.[89] More specifically, epidemics of influenza have been linked with the excess of cardiovascular deaths during the winter.[90] However, the risk attributable to influenza outside such epidemic periods is probably low, and evidence for a direct role for this infection in acute coronary syndromes is lacking.

Further evidence for the potential influence of respiratory infection in CHD comes from a prospective case–control study of 150 consecutive patients admitted to hospital with MI, who were matched for age, gender and admission date with 150 hospital controls (without cardiorespiratory disease).[91] Common cold or flu-like symptoms in the 2 weeks preceding admission had occurred in 42 (28%) of the cases and 23 (15%) of the controls (odds ratio 2.2). It is possible that such illnesses lead to pro-atherogenic inflammatory changes. In keeping with this idea, a prospective study in the UK involving 96 people (aged 65–74 years) found that serum fibrinogen (and factor VIIc) levels tended to be higher in the winter compared with other seasons and correlated with elevated neutrophil counts, CRP and self-reported cough and coryzal symptoms.[88] The researchers suggested that minor respiratory infections might have activated acute phase reactants and hence accounted for the raised fibrinogen levels, and contributed to the excess cardiovascular risk in winter months.

One case-contol study involving 9571 patients (1922 cases diagnosed with acute MI; 7649 age- and sex-matched controls) found significantly more cases than controls had an acute respiratory infection in the 10 days before the cardiac event (2.8% versus 0.9%, relative risk for MI 2.7 [1.6–4.7]).[92] No increase in MI rates was found in relation to urinary tract infections. Adjustments were made in this study for smoking status and body mass index (BMI) but not for social class. The investigators speculated that acute respiratory infections might be a trigger of acute MI, with systemic inflammation (secondary to the infection) leading to increasing levels of CRP, fibrinogen and cytokines. Such changes might, in turn, increase any tendency towards plaque instability and rupture with subsequent thrombosis.

Coxsachievirus B infections

A few studies have suggested an association between coxsachievirus B infection and acute MI. For example, coxsachievirus B-specific IgM responses were measured in 329 patients admitted to a single coronary care unit over a 12-month period and compared with serum responses in 178 age-matched controls.[93] Patients with acute MI were observed to be significantly more likely to have positive seropositivity to coxsachievirus B-specific IgM than the controls (p=0.02). Other studies have failed to demonstrate such an association[94] and overall, the data remain inconsistent. No prospective cohort study has been performed. There is a much clearer correlation between acute myocarditis and coxsachievirus B infection.[95]

Enterovirus infections

An association between enterovirus infections and the risk of MI has been reported.[96] In a prospective, nested case–control study, higher levels of anti-enterovirus (ECV) antibodies were significantly associated with developing MI in middle-aged men (n=183 cases; n=228 controls, 9-year follow-up). Among women, there was a trend towards higher levels of anti-ECV antibodies in those who had gone on to develop MI, but this was not statistically significant. Interestingly, no differences were found between cases and controls (men or women) in their levels of antibodies to heat-denatured coxsackievirus B5 or adenovirus hexon protein. The investigators acknowledged that it remains unclear whether higher levels of ECV reflect a history of frequent ECV infections (and which may be a risk factor for MI), whether genetic factors predisposing to MI also predispose to enhanced serum antibody responses, or whether ECV antibody levels are simply based on cross-reactions with host-cell proteins.

HIV infection

Paton *et al.* described a series of eight HIV-positive males whose autopsies revealed marked atherosclerotic changes in the coronary arteries.[97] The lesions were unusual for healthy subjects in this age group (23–32 years) without typical atherogenic risk factors. The authors concluded that viral infection (either HIV or co-existing herpesviruses) had probably contributed to the development of the coronary artery pathology. In another autopsy study, distinctive pathological changes (intimal elastosis and medial dysplasia) in the coronary arteries were more frequently found in 32 male patients (mean age, 41 years) with HIV than in a similar number of age-matched controls.[98] There was, however, no signficant difference in the prevalence of cardiovascular risk factors or in the incidence and severity of clinically overt CHD between the two groups of patients.

What about *C. pneumoniae?*

There is a lack of evidence to suggest that any of the organisms discussed above have a causal role in CHD. In particular, relevant prospective data are either limited or absent. By contrast, there is a large and growing body of research implicating the intracellular pathogen, *C. pneumoniae,* with atherogenesis. This evidence includes data from sero-epidemiological studies, direct examination of atherosclerotic plaques, animal models and preliminary clinical intervention studies.

These findings (to be reviewed in later chapters) make *C. pneumoniae* a far more plausible potential contributor to the pathogenesis of atherosclerotic disease than any of the other microorganisms so far discussed.

Summary

Common chronic infections may contribute to atherogenesis and CHD progression. It is now generally accepted that atherosclerosis has an inflammatory component but whether antigens from microorganisms represent the trigger or are modulating factors of such inflammation is unclear. Overall, prospective and longitudinal data are either limited or absent for most of the infections discussed in this chapter. CMV infections seem to be associated with the development of coronary artery restenosis and/or graft vasculopathy (rather than 'native' atherosclerosis). In the case of *H. pylori,* the presence of confounding factors (principally socioeconomic class) seems to preclude any independent link with CHD, although stronger evidence suggests that the more virulent Cag-A strain may have relevant pro-inflammatory and possibly pro-atherogenic effects. Evidence linking chronic dental sepsis and respiratory infections with CHD is intriguing, but certainly not conclusive.

Chlamydia pneumoniae is currently the leading potential 'culprit' infection in CHD. The next chapter outlines the epidemiology and microbiology of this organism. Much of the remainder of the book reviews evidence implicating *C. pneumoniae* in atherosclerosis and CHD, and discusses how the organism might trigger or promote such disease.

References

1. Osler W. Diseases of the arteries. In: *Modern Medicine: Its Practice and Theory* (Osler W, ed.). Lea & Febiger, Philadephia, USA, 1908; pp. 429–47.
2. Nieminen MS, Mattila K, Valtonen V. Infection and inflammation as risk factors for myocardial infarction. *Eur Heart J* 1993; **14**(Suppl. K): 12–6.
3. Buja LM. Does atherosclerosis have an infectious etiology? *Circulation* 1996; **94**: 872–3.
4. Hennekens CH. Increasing burden of cardiovascular disease: current knowledge and future directions for research on risk factors. *Circulation* 1998; **97**: 1095–102.
5. Gupta S, Camm AJ. Is there an infective aetiology to atherosclerosis? *Drugs Aging* 1998; **13**: 1–7.
6. Ridker PM. Inflammation, infection and cardiovascular risk: How good is the clinical evidence? *Circulation* 1998; **97**: 1671–4.
7. Marshall BJ. *Helicobacter pylori* in peptic ulcer: Have Koch's postulates been fulfilled? *Ann Med* 1995; **27**: 565–8.
8. Silman AJ. Is rheumatoid arthritis an infectious disease? *BMJ* 1991; **303**: 200–1.
9. Sanderson JD, Moss MT, Tizard ML, Hermon-Taylor J. *Mycobacterium paratuberculosis* DNA in Crohn's disease tissues. *Gut* 1992; **33**: 890–6.
10. Soldan SS, Bertri R, Salem N *et al.* Association of human herpes virus 6 (HHV-6) with multiple sclerosis: increased IgG response to HHV-6 early antigen and detection of serum HHV-6 DNA. *Nature Medicine* 1998; **3**: 1394–7.
11. Saboor SA, Johnson N, McFadden J. Detection of mycobacterial DNA in sarcoidosis and tuberculosis with polymerase chain reaction. *Lancet* 1992; **339**: 1012–5.
12. Ross R. The pathogenesis of atherosclerosis: a perspective for the 1990s. *Nature* 1993; **362**: 801–9.
13. Ho DD, Rota TR, Andrews CA, Hirsch MS. Replication of human cytomegalovirus in endothelial cells. *J Infect Dis* 1984; **150**: 956–7.
14. Hajjar DP. Viral pathogenesis of atherosclerosis. *Am J Pathol* 1991; **139**: 1195–210.
15. Kirkpatrick CJ, Bultmann BD, Gruler H. Interaction between enteroviruses and human endothelial cells *in vitro*. Alterations in the physical properties of endothelial cell plasma membrane and adhesion of human granulocytes. *Am J Pathol* 1985; **118**: 15–25.
16. Kaukoranta-Tolvanen SS, Laitinen K, Saikku P, Leinonen M. *Chlamydia pneumoniae* multiplies in human endothelial cells *in vitro*. *Microbial Pathog* 1994; **16**: 313–9.
17. Reidy MA, Bowyer DE. Distortion of endothelial repair. The effect of hypercholesterolemia on regulation of aortic endothelium following injury by endotoxin. A scanning microscopy study. *Atherosclerosis* 1978; **29**: 459–66.
18. Pesonen E, Kaprio E, Rapola J, Soveri T, Oksanen H. Endothelial cell damage in piglet coronary artery after administration of *E. coli* endotoxin. A scanning and transmission electron-microscopic study. *Atherosclerosis* 1981; **40**: 65–73.
19. Hansson GK, Jonasson L, Seifert PS, Stemme S. Immune mechanisms in atherosclerosis. *Arteriosclerosis* 1989; **9**: 567–78.
20. Etingin OR, Hajjar DP. Evidence for cytokine regulation of cholesterol metabolism in herpesvirus-infected arterial cells by the lipoxygenase pathway. *J Lipid Res* 1990; **31**: 299–305.
21. Hajjar DP, Falcone DJ, Fabricant CG, Fabricant J. Altered cholesteryl ester cycle is associated with lipid accumulation in herpesvirus-infected arterial smooth muscle cells. *J Biol Chem* 1985; **260**: 6124–8.
22. Leatham EW, Bath PM, Tooze JA, Camm AJ. Increased monocyte tissue factor expression in coronary disease. *Br Heart J* 1995; **73**: 10–13.
23. Visser MR, Tracey PB, Vercellottii GM *et al.* Enhanced thrombin generation and platelet binding on herpes simplex virus-infected endothelium. *Proc Natl Acad Sci USA* 1988; **85**: 8227–30.

24. Paterson J, Cottral GE. Experimental coronary sclerosis. Lymphomatosis as a cause of coronary sclerosis in chickens. *Arch Pathol* 1950; **49**: 699.
25. Fabricant CG, Fabricant J, Litrenta MM, Minick CR. Virus-induced atherosclerosis. *J Exp Med* 1978; **148**: 335–40.
26. Fabricant CG, Fabricant J, Minick CR, Litrenta MM. Herpesvirus-induced atherosclerosis in chickens. *Fed Proc* 1983; **42**: 2467–9.
27. Minick CR, Fabricant CG, Fabricant J, Litrenta MM. Atheroarteriosclerosis induced by infection with a herpesvirus. *Am J Path* 1979; **96**: 673–706.
28. Fabricant CG, Hajjar DP, Minick CR, Fabricant J. Herpesvirus infcetion enhances cholesterol and cholesteryl ester accumulation in cultured arterial smooth muscle cells. *Am J Path* 1981; **105**: 176–84.
29. Pyrzak R, Shih JC. Detection of specific DNA segments of Marek's disease herpes virus in quail susceptible to atherosclerosis. *Atherosclerosis* 1987; **68**: 77–85.
30. Span AH, Grauls G, Bosman F, Van Boven CP, Bruggeman CA. Cytomegalovirus infection induces vascular injury in the rat. *Artherosclerosis* 1992; **93**: 41–52.
31. Lemstrom KB, Bruning JH, Bruggeman CA *et al.* Cytomegalovirus infection enhances smooth muscle cell proliferation and intimal thickening of rat aortic allograft. *J Clin Invest* 1993; **92**: 549–58.
32. Melnick JL, Adam E, Debakey ME. Cytomegalovirus and atherosclerosis. *Eur Heart J* 1993; **14** (Suppl K): 30–8.
33. Melnick JL, Petrie BL, Dreesman GR *et al.* Cytomegalovirus antigen within human arterial smooth muscle cells. *Lancet* 1983; **2**: 644–7.
34. Gyorkey F, Melnick JL, Guinn GA, Gyorkey P, DeBakey ME. Herpesviridae in the endothelial and smooth muscle cells of the proximal aorta in arteriosclerotic patients. *Exp Mol Pathol* 1984; **40**: 328–39.
35. Hendrix MG, Dormans PH, Kitslaar P, Bosman F, Bruggeman CA. The presence of cytomegalovirus nucleic acids in arterial walls of atherosclerotic and non-atherosclerotic patients. *Am J Pathol* 1989; **134**: 1151–7.
36. Hendrix MG, Salimans MM, van Boven CP, Bruggeman CA. High prevalence of latently present cytomegalovirus in arterial walls of patients suffering from grade III atherosclerosis. *Am J Pathol* 1990; **136**: 23–8.
37. Hendrix MG, Daemen M, Bruggeman CA. Cytomegalovirus nucleic acid distribution within the human vascular tree. *Am J Pathol* 1991; **138**: 563–7.
38. Bruggeman CA, Dam-Mieras MC. The possible role of cytomegalovirus in atherogenesis. In: *Progress in Medical Virology* (Melnick JL, ed) vol 38. Karger, Basel, Switzerland, 1991; pp. 1–26.
39. Yamashiroya HM, Ghosh L, Yang R, Robertson AL Jr. Herpesviridae in the coronary arteries and aorta of young trauma victims. *Am J Pathol* 1988; **130**: 71–9.
40. Danesh J, Collins R, Peto R. Chronic infections and coronary heart disease: is there a link? *Lancet* 1997; **350**: 430–6.
41. Adam E, Melnick JL, Probtsfield JL *et al.* High levels of cytomegalovirus antibody in patients requiring vascular surgery for atherosclerosis. *Lancet* 1987; **2**: 291–3.
42. Melnick SL, Shahar E, Folsom AR *et al.* Past infection by *Chlamydia pneumoniae* strain TWAR and asymptomatic carotid atherosclerosis. Atherosclerosis Risk in Communities (ARIC) Study Investigators. *Am J Med* 1993; **95**: 499–504.
43. Heiss G, Sharrett AR, Barnes R *et al.* Carotid atherosclerosis measured by B-mode ultrasound in populations: associations with cardiovascular risk factors in the ARIC Study. *Am J Epidemiol* 1991; **134**: 250–6.
44. Sorlie PD, Adam E, Melnick JL *et al.* Cytomegalovirus/herpesvirus and carotid atherosclerosis: the ARIC study. *J Med Virol* 1994; **42**: 33–7.
45. Nieto FJ, Adam E, Sorlie P *et al.* Cohort study of cytomegalovirus infection as a risk factor for carotid intimal-medial thickening, a measure of subclinical atherosclerosis. *Circulation* 1996; **94**: 922–7.

46. Alder SP, Hur JK, Wang JB *et al.* Prior infection with cytomegalovirus is not a major risk factor for angiographically demonstrated coronary artery atherosclerosis. *J Infect Dis* 1998; **177**: 209–12.
47. Chiu B, Viira E, Tucker W, Fong IA. *Chlamydia pneumoniae*, cytomegalovirus, and herpes simplex virus in atherosclerosis of the carotid artery. *Circulation* 1997; **96**: 2144–8.
48. Speir E, Modali R, Huang ES *et al.* Potential role of human cytomegalovirus and p53 interaction in coronary restenosis. *Science* 1994; **265**: 391–4.
49. Zhou YF, Leon MB, Waclawiw MA. Association between prior cytomegalovirus infection and the risk of restenosis after coronary atherectomy. *N Engl J Med* 1996; **335**: 624–30.
50. Radke PW, Merkelbach S, Dörge H *et al.* Low frequency of detectable human cytomegalovirus DNA in coronary atherosclerotic lesions obtained by coronary endatherectomy. *J Am Coll Cardiol* 1998; **271-A**: 1111–31[abstract].
51. Kol A, Sperti G, Shani J *et al.* Cytomegalovirus replication is not a cause of instability in unstable angina. *Circulation* 1995; **91**: 1910–3.
52. Grattan MT, Moreno-Cabral CE, Starnes VA *et al.* Cytomegalovirus infection is associated with cardiac allograft rejection and atherosclerosis. *JAMA* 1989; **261**: 3561–6.
53. Johnson DE, Gao SZ, Schroeder JS, DeCampli WM, Billingham ME. The spectrum of coronary artery pathological findings in human cardiac allografts. *J Heart Transplant* 1989; **8**: 349–59.
54. Grattan MT. Accelerated graft atherosclerosis following cardiac transplantation: Clinical perspectives. *Clin Cardiol* 1991; **14** (Suppl II): 16–20.
55. McDonald K, Rector TS, Braunlin EA, Kubo SH, Olirari MT. Association of coronary artery disease in cardiac transplant recipients with cytomegalovirus infection. *Am J Cardiol* 1989; **64**: 359–62.
56. Wu TC, Hruban RH, Ambinder RF *et al.* Demonstration of cytomegalovirus nucleic acids in the coronary arteries of transplanted hearts. *Am J Pathol* 1992; **140**: 739–47.
57. Libby P, Egan D, Skarlatos S. Roles of infectious agents in atherosclerosis and restenosis: an assessment of the current evidence and need for future research. *Circulation* 1997; **96**: 4095–103.
58. Key NS, Vercellotti GM, Winkelmann JC *et al.* Infection of vascular endothelial cells with herpes simplex virus enhances tissue factor activity and reduces thrombomodulin expression. *Proc Natl Acad Sci USA* 1990; **87**: 7095–9.
59. Etingin OR, Silverstein RL, Hajjar DP. Identification of monocyte receptor on herpes-infected endothelial cells. *Proc Natl Acad Sci USA* 1991; **88**: 7200–3.
60. Dummer S, Lee A, Breinig MK *et al.* Investigation of cytomegalovirus infection as a risk factor for coronary atherosclerosis in the explanted hearts of patients undergoing heart transplantation. *J Med Virol* 1994; **44**: 305–9.
61. Mendall MA, Goggin P, Molineaux N *et al.* Childhood living conditions and *Helicobacter* seropositivity in adult life. *Lancet* 1992; **i**: 896–7.
62. Langman MJ, Cooke AR. Gastric and duodenal ulcer and their associated diseases. *Lancet* 1976; **i**: 680–3.
63. Mendall MA, Goggin PM, Molineaux N *et al.* Relation of *Helicobacter pylori* infection and coronary heart disease. *Br Heart J* 1994; **71**: 437–9.
64. Patel P, Mendall MA, Carrington D *et al.* Association of *Helicobacter pylori* and *Chlamydia pneumoniae* infections with coronary heart disease and cardiovascular risk factors. *BMJ* 1995; **311**: 711–4.
65. Birnie DH, Holme ER, McKay IC *et al.* Association between antibodies to heat shock protein 65 and coronary atherosclerosis. *Eur Heart J* 1998; **19**: 387–94.
66. Parente F, Maconi G, Imbesi V *et al. Helicobacter pylori* infection and coagulation in healthy people. *BMJ* 1997; **314**: 1318–9.
67. Murray LJ, Bamford KB, O'Reilly DP, McCrum EE, Evans AE. *Helicobacter pylori* infection: relation with cardiovascular risk factors, ischaemic heart disease, and social class. *Br Heart J* 1995; **74**: 497–501.

68. Whincup PH, Mendall MA, Perry I, Strachan DP, Walker M. Prospective relations between *Helicobacter pylori* infection, coronary heart disease and stroke in middle aged men. *Heart* 1996; **75**: 568–72.
69. Wald NJ, Law MR, Morris JK, Bagnall AM. *Helicobacter pylori* infection and mortality from ischaemic heart disease: negative results from a large, prospective study. *BMJ* 1997; **315**: 1199–201.
70. Strandberg TE, Tilvis RS, Vuoristo M, Lindroos M, Kosunen TU. Prospective study of *Helicobacter pylori* seropositivity and cardiovascular diseases in a general elderly population. *BMJ* 1997; **314**: 1317–8.
71. Strachan DP, Mendall MA, Carrington D *et al.* Relation of *Helicobacter pylori* infection to 13-year mortality and incident ischemic heart disease in the Caerphilly prospective heart disease study. *Circulation* 1998; **98**: 1286–90.
72. Sandifer QD, Vuilo S, Crompton G. Association of *Helicobacter pylori* infection with coronary heart disease: association may not be causal. *BMJ* 1996; **312**: 251 [letter].
73. Danesh J, Peto R. Risk factors for coronary heart disease and infection with *Helicobacter pylori*: meta-analysis of 18 studies. *BMJ* 1998; **316**: 1130–2.
74. Blasi F, Denti F, Erba M *et al.* Detection of *Chlamydia pneumoniae* but not *Helicobacter pylori* in atherosclerotic plaques of aortic aneurysms. *J Clin Microbiol* 1996; **34**: 2766–9.
75. Pasceri V, Cammarota G, Patti G *et al.* Association of virulent *Helicobacter pylori* strains with ischemic heart disease. *Circulation* 1998; **97**: 1675–9.
76. Loesche WJ. Role of *Streptococcus mutans* in human dental decay. *Microbiol Rev* 1986; **50**: 353–80.
77. Slots J, Listgarten MA. *Bacteroides gingivalis*, *Bacteroides intermedius* and *Actinobacillus actinomycetemcomitans* in human periodontal diseases. *J Clin Periodontol* 1988; **15**: 85–93.
78. Mackenzie RS, Millard HD. Interrelated effects of diabetes, arteriosclerosis and calculus on alveolar bone loss. *J Am Dent Assoc* 1963; **66**: 192–8.
79. Syrjänen J, Peltola J, Valtonen V *et al.* Dental infections in association with cerebral infarction in young and middle-aged men. *J Intern Med* 1989; **225**: 179–84.
80. Mattila K, Nieminen M, Valtonen V *et al.* Association between dental health and acute myocardial infarction. *BMJ* 1989; **298**: 779–82.
81. Paunio K, Impivaara O, Tickso J, Maki J. Missing teeth and ischaemic heart disease in men aged 45–64 years. *Eur Heart J* 1993; **14** (Suppl K): 54–6.
82. Mattila K, Valle MS, Nieminen MS, Valtonen VV, Hietanieni KL. Dental infections and coronary atherosclerosis. *Atherosclerosis* 1993; **103**: 205–11.
83. Seymour RA, Steele JG. Is there a link between periodontal disease and coronary heart disease? *Br Dent J* 1998; **184**: 33–8.
84. Kweider M, Lowe GD, Murray GD, Kinane DF, McGowen DA. Dental disease, fibrinogen and white cell counts: links with myocardial infarction? *Scot Med J* 1993; **38**: 73–4.
85. Mattila K, Rasi V, Nieminen MS *et al.* Von Willebrand factor antigen and dental infections. *Thromb Res* 1989; **56**: 325–9.
86. Shapira L, Soskolne WA, Sela MN, Offenbacher S, Barak V. The secretion of PGE_2, IL-1 beta, IL-6 and TNF-alpha by adherent mononuclear cells from early onset periodontitis patients. *J Periodontol* 1994; **65**: 139–46.
87. Marchant B, Ranjadayalan K, Stevenson R, Wilkinson P, Timmis AD. Circadian and seasonal factors in the pathogenesis of acute myocardial infarction: the influence of environmental temperature. *Br Heart J* 1993; **69**: 385–7.
88. Woodhouse PR, Khaw TK, Plummer M, Foley A, Meade TW. Seasonal variations of plasma fibrinogen and factor VII activity in the elderly: winter infections and deaths from cardiovascular disease. *Lancet* 1994; **343**: 435–9.
89. Enquselassie F, Dobson AJ, Alexander HM, Steele PL. Seasons, temperature and coronary disease. *Int J Epidemiol* 1993; **22**: 632–6.
90. Housworth J, Langmuir AD. Excess mortality from epidemic influenza, 1957–1966. *Am J Epidemiol* 1974; **100**: 40–8.

91. Spodick DH, Flessas AP, Johnson MM. Association of acute respiratory symptoms with onset of acute myocardial infarction: prospective investigation of 150 consecutive patients and matched controls. *Am J Cardiol* 1984; **53**: 481–2.
92. Meier CR, Jick SS, Derby LE, Vasilakis C, Jick H. Acute respiratory-tract infections and risk of first-time acute myocardial infarction. *Lancet* 1998; **351**: 1467–8.
93. Lau RC. Coxsackie B virus-specific IgM responses in coronary care unit patients. *J Med Virol* 1986; **18**: 193–8.
94. Hannington G, Booth JC, Bowes RJ, Stern JC. Coxsackie B virus-specific IgM antibody and myocardial infarction. *J Med Microbiol* 1986; **21**: 287–91.
95. Levi G, Scalvini S, Volterrani M *et al.* Coxsackie virus heart disease. *Eur Heart J* 1988; **9**: 1303–7.
96. Roivainen M, Alfthan G, Jousilahti P *et al.* Enterovirus infections as a possible risk factor for myocardial infarction. *Circulation* 1998; **98**: 2534–7.
97. Paton P, Tabib A, Loire R, Tete R. Coronary artery lesions and human immunodeficiency virus infection. *Res Virol* 1993; **144**: 225–31.
98. Best PJM, Edwards WD, Holmes Jr DR, Lerman A. Unique coronary arteriopathy associated with human immunodeficiency virus. *J Am Coll Cardiol* 1998; **272A**: 1111–32 [abstract].

Chapter 3: *Chlamydia pneumoniae*: Natural history, epidemiology and microbiology

Introduction

Chlamydia pneumoniae is a very common cause of infection in humans. Before reviewing evidence implicating *C. pneumoniae* in atherogenesis, it is worth considering background details on the organism itself. Of particular relevance are the natural history, epidemiology and microbiology of *C. pneumoniae* and other chalmydial species, and available anti-chlamydial antibiotic treatments.

Background

Chlamydiae are obligate intracellular parasites. They cannot synthesise adenosine triphosphate or guanosine triphosphate, and so depend wholly on energy produced by the host cell. In some respects, they resemble large viruses. However, the presence of a Lipopolysacchoride (LPS) cell wall, DNA and RNA, and the ability of the organisms to replicate by binary fission classifies them as Gram-negative bacteria.[1] There are three main species of Chlamydiae: *Chlamydia trachomatis* and *C. pneumoniae* are primarily pathogens of man; *Chlamydia psittaci* mainly infects birds. *Chlamydia pecorum* infects sheep and cattle and, so far, has not been described in humans.[2]

Range of infection in humans

Chlamydial infection is a major cause of disease in humans.[3] Trachoma (caused by *C. trachomatis* infection) is the leading preventable cause of blindness in the world.[4] Genital *C. trachomatis* is the principal cause of pelvic inflammatory disease in the UK and the USA,[5] and of neonatal inclusion conjunctivitis worldwide.[6]

Chlamydia pneumoniae species was first identified as a respiratory pathogen in 1986.[7] (See Figure 5.) As early as 1943, Smadel had described cases of *Chlamydia*-induced pneumonia in humans who had had no prior contact with birds (as reviewed by Allegra, 1995),[8] which are potential sources of *C. psittaci*. Later, an 'atypical' *C. psittaci* strain was found to be responsible for acute respiratory infections in young adults.[7,9] This strain was given the name TWAR, an acronym generated from the names of two early isolates: TW-183 (isolated in 1965 from the conjunctiva of a child during a trachoma vaccine study in Taiwan) and AR-39 (isolated in 1983 from a throat swab of a student in Seattle).[7]

Figure 5: Fluorescence micrograph of McCoy cells inoculated with *C. pneumonaie*

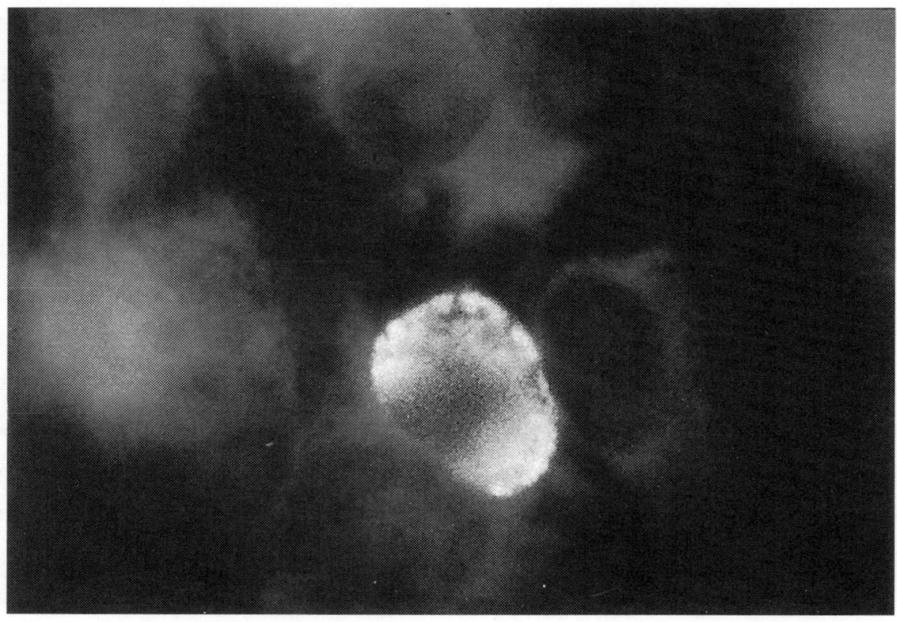

Natural history of Chlamydiae

Life cycle

The interaction between chlamydiae and their host cells includes several distinct stages:

- Attachment to and entry into host cells
- Parasitism of host cell's energy supply
- Chlamydial reproductive cycle within cells
- Persistence of chlamydial infections in some cells
- Cell destruction with liberation of new infective particles

Chlamydiae exist in two distinct forms in their life developmental cycle – infectious elementary bodies and larger non-infectious reproductive reticulate bodies. The 'pear-shaped' elementary bodies infect host cells, probably via a receptor-mediated process.[10] Elements of the chlamydial cell wall, which is composed of outer and inner membrane proteins and LPS (the genus-specific antigen[11,12]) probably facilitate attachment of infectious chlamydial organisms to host cells. In keeping with this idea, the major outer membrane protein (MOMP) contains several highly cross-reactive proteins that may help reduce the mutual electrostatic repulsion that usually occurs between host cells and elementary bodies.[13] Having entered host cells, elementary bodies differentiate into reticulate bodies, which then multiply intracellularly, using the host's supply of energy and nutrients. The endotoxin activity of chlamydial LPS seems to be much lower than that of LPS from Gram-negative enterobacteria.[14] Chlamydial LPS is, therefore, less likely than those of other microorganisms to trigger the host's immune defences and so may allow chlamydiae to establish long-lasting parasitic relationships with the host.[15] At the same time, MOMP and other antigens are released on to the host cell surfaces and can thereby stimulate neutralising antibody responses. The reticulate bodies convert to elementary bodies by processes of re-organisation and condensation.[16] The developmental cycle normally (but not necessarily) ends in rupture of the host cell with release of thousands of elementary bodies that can then initiate a new cycle in adjacent cells.[17]

Immunopathological consequences

Chlamydial infections are usually limited temporally by potent cell-mediated and humoral immune responses. However, such infections do not elicit any long-lasting immune protection from reinfection. Immunity is only partial and short-lived, and re-infections are common.[18] In a persistent infection, continual re-exposure to the organism may lead to hypersensitivity reactions with associated tissue injury. During this phase, features of inflammation are prominent but chlamydial organisms are rarely isolated.[19] The significance of hypersensitivity responses in chronic chlamydial infections first emerged in 1962 during anti-chlamydial vaccination trials in humans and primates.[20] Prior immunisation with killed chlamydial organisms led to a more severe disease during infection, suggesting that the immunisation primed the host to develop a deleterious hypensensitivity response.

It has been suggested that the immunopathological sequelae of chronic chlamydial infections may be mediated via release of so-called heat shock (or stress) proteins (HSPs).[21] These proteins have important functions in cellular metabolism and help cells to deal with adverse environmental stimuli.[22] HSPs are induced in cells by several factors such as heat, acute or chronic infection and other unfavourable conditions. They are highly conserved, and HSPs from eukaryotic cells, parasites and bacteria exhibit wide cross-reactivity.[23] Recent studies have shown that Chlamydiae possess at least two HSPs: the 60 kD and the 70 kD protein.[24,25]

Epidemiology of *C. pneumoniae*

Chlamydia pneumoniae usually causes around 6–10% of cases of community-acquired pneumonia.[26,27] However, during epidemics, it may account for 50% of such infections worldwide.[28] Most acute chlamydial infections are subclinical or produce only mild flu-like symptoms,[9] or pharyngitis, otitis media or sinusitis;[29] only rarely does the organism cause life-threatening infections.[30]

Chlamydia pneumoniae infection spreads via respiratory droplets. Studies in families and military recruits suggest that the infection has an incubation period of 3–4 weeks.[31,32] Interestingly, however, anti-*C. pneumoniae* antibody prevalence appears unusually low among certain remote African tribes,[33] in which the population density seems too low for there to be continuous circulation of the organism. Population data accumulated from all age groups in Seattle, USA shows that the prevalence of anti-*C. pneumoniae* IgG antibodies is low in those aged under 5 years, but then increases rapidly with age until about 15 years and then more slowly throughout the rest of life, reaching about 70% in older adults.[32] Around 50% of middle-aged adults worldwide have antibodies to *C. pneumoniae*.[30,34] The antibody prevalence in males is generally 20–25% higher than in females,[26] perhaps due to the higher rates of smoking and related respiratory infection among men.

Given that the anti-*C. pneumoniae* antibody titre usually falls with eventual loss of measurable antibody 3–5 years after infection, the population prevalence data suggest that reinfection is common. Overall, most people probably have two or three *C. pneumoniae* infections during their lifetime.[25]

Chronic *C. pneumoniae* infection

A major element in *C. pneumoniae*'s role as a human pathogen is its ability to persist within the body and cause chronic infections. (In general, the terms 'chronic', 'latent' and 'persistent' are used interchangeably in relation to chlamydial infection.) Whether the chlamydial antigens change during infection such that they become less easily recognised by the immune system, or whether other factors allow the organism to persist, is unclear.[10] The infection has been linked with several chronic inflammatory conditions, in particular, coronary heart disease (CHD) and atherosclerosis. (See Table 3.) Case study reports provide some very limited and debatable evidence of associations between *C. pneumoniae* and sarcoidosis,[35] reactive arthritis[36] and Guillain–Barré syndrome.[37] There is also evidence to suggest that chronic *C. pneumoniae* infection exacerbates wheezing episodes in asthma[38] and bronchitis.[39] In addition, some investigators have suggested *C. pneumoniae* infections may partly explain the increased incidence of asthma seen over recent years in many countries.[40]

Table 3: *Chlamydia pneumoniae* and its association with chronic diseases

Asthma
Sarcoidosis
Arthritis
Guillain–Barré
Lung Cancer
Atherosclerosis

Repeated exposure to *C. trachomatis* antigen(s) in the course of chronic infections is central to the development of both scarring trachoma and fallopian tube obstruction,[41] processes which probably involves a hypersensitivity reaction to chlamydial HSP 60.[42] Whether similar mechanisms exist in persistent *C. pneumoniae* infection is not known.

Diagnosis of *C. pneumoniae* infection

Traditionally, the laboratory diagnosis of any infection is made by the identification of the microorganism by culture techniques applied to specimens taken from symptomatic patients, or, in some cases, by the detection of an antibody response to the organism.

Diagnosis of acute *C. pneumoniae* infection is difficult.[43] Four main diagnostic techniques have been tried, with varying degrees of success (see Table 4). Establishing whether or not persistent *C. pneumoniae* infection is a cause of chronic disease is even more difficult. A fundamental diagnostic problem lies in determining whether or not the pathogen triggers an abnormal self-perpetuating reaction that causes progression of disease (such as atherosclerosis), while *C. pneumoniae* itself becomes latent or disappears.

Table 4: Some laboratory methods applied in the diagnosis of *C. pneumoniae* infection

Isolation in cell culture
HeLa 229 cell cultures
Hep 2 cell cultures
McCoy cell cultures
Antigen detection
Direct immunofluorescence test
Enzyme immunoassay
Serological antibody tests
Complement fixation test
Microimmunofluorescence test
Polymerase chain reaction

Microbiological culture

Chlamydia pneumoniae has proved difficult to isolate, even in acute infection. Also, where chronic infection is suspected, a negative result in an isolation test is not a reliable indicator of the organism's absence. Attempts to propagate the organism in culture have been largely unsuccessful despite use of several well-established cell lines (e.g. HeLa 229 or Hep 2). The organism grows poorly in comparison with the other chlamydial species. In addition, *C. pneumoniae* organisms are susceptible to destruction by techniques that involve a freeze–thaw cycle: rapid freezing inactivates more than 50% of the organisms.[29] Of interest, although *C. trachomatis* is relatively easy to culture in the setting of acute infections, cell culture studies are rarely positive in chronic *C. trachomatis* infections.[44]

Serological tests

In the case of *C. trachomatis* and *C. psittaci*, the MOMPs (encoded by the omp1 gene[45]) contain species-specific antigens and, therefore, allow differentiation between these species by serological methods using microimmunofluorescence techniques based on anti-MOMP monoclonal antibodies. By contrast, the 39.5 kD MOMP antigen of *C. pneumoniae* shows cross-reactivity with other chlamydial species.[34] This antigen is easily destroyed by physical or chemical treatment, and this has hindered efforts to characterise it.[46]

Microimmunofluorescence test

The type-specific microimmunofluorescence test (originally devised in 1970 for *C. trachomatis*[47]) remains the only specific and sensitive serological test for detecting evidence of *C. pneumoniae* infection. This test allows differentiation of IgM, IgA and IgG antibodies, potentially allowing the recognition of both current and previous infections, and commonly uses fixed whole elementary bodies as antigen; the target epitopes probably reside on the MOMP. The microimmunofluorescence test, when read by an experienced microscopist, can distinguish reliably between specific reactions and various 'noises' from cross-reacting antibodies to other chlamydial or bacterial species.[48] The test does not give an exact numerical value and, in terms of consistency, depends on the reliability of the microscope and reagents, as well as the experience of the reader. As yet, there is no standardised quality control system to check performance of the microimmunofluorescence test in different laboratories.

A preliminary report has shown a relatively low inter-laboratory variability in the results of microimmunofluorescence assays used in serodiagnosis of *C. pneumoniae* infection.[49] Although the absolute values for IgG and IgM responses to *C. pneumoniae* infection varied from laboratory to laboratory, the overall agreement of all 14 participating laboratories (with a 'gold standard' set from the central laboratory in Washington DC, USA) was 80% (range 60–90%). Although encouraged by the findings, the authors acknowledge that further studies are needed to define the factors that require standardisation for these assays.

Suggested criteria for positive antibody tests are shown in Table 5.

Table 5: Serological diagnosis of *C. pneumoniae* infection

Acute infection
fourfold IgG titre rise
Single IgM titre ≥1/16
Single IgG titre ≥1/512
Pre-existing/chronic infection
IgG titre ≥1/16 and ≤1/512

Complement fixation tests

Complement fixation tests rely on serum antibodies interacting with the chlamydial genus LPS antigen. Since this antigen is shared by all chlamydial organisms, the test cannot differentiate between chlamydial species.[43] Accordingly, it is now clear that many patients diagnosed as having 'psittacosis' (presumed to be caused by *C. psittaci*) on the basis of a positive complement fixation test results were, in reality, infected with *C. pneumoniae*. The complement fixation test is positive in under one-third of patients with other evidence of exposure to *C. pneumoniae* infection, and older patients may not show a positive complement fixation test response (despite having other evidence of *C. pneumoniae* infection).[26]

Enzyme-linked immunosorbent assay tests

The microimmunofluorescence assay is generally accepted as the gold standard for the serological diagnosis of an acute *C. pneumoniae* infection. However, interpretation of specific and non-specific fluorescence patterns requires considerable expertise and cross-reactions may occur with other chlamydial species. Partly as a result of such factors, an increasing role may emerge for enzyme-linked immunoabsorbent assay (ELISA) detection of anti-chlamydial antibodies. Chemically pure antigens have been isolated for the detection of antibodies against chlamydial LPS; this has led to the development of a commercially available recombinant DNA LPS ELISA.[50] In a study by Verkooyen *et al.*, the rDNA LPS ELISA appeared to be a more sensitive detector of acute respiratory chlamydial infection than was the traditional microimmunofluorescence methods, and demonstrated a high degree of reproducibility.[51] However, a major limitation is that the ELISA test is genus- and not species-specific.

Serology and infection status

Antibody prevalence studies in industrialised countries have shown that among the general population, of the different chlamydial species, IgG antibodies against *C. pneumoniae* are by far the most common and tend to be found in the highest titres.[52] In addition, anti-*C. pneumoniae* antibody titre levels measured using microimmunofluorescence are often comparable with anti-*C. trachomatis* antibody titres found in infertile women with chronic pelvic inflammatory disease, or in men or women with lymphogranuloma venerum.[52] These titre levels can be explained partly by booster effects caused by re-infections, but may also suggest the existence of chronic *C. pneumoniae* infection analogous to persistent, deep-sited *C. trachomatis* infections. Despite such evidence, serology is a controversial indicator of chronic *C. pneumoniae* infection. First, it gives no indication of the site of a such infection. Secondly, anti-*C. pneumoniae* antibodies are so common (especially in older age groups) that proving an association with a specific disease (such as CHD) is difficult. Thirdly, epidemics might temporarily induce high antibody titres in control populations. Despite these limitations, a continuously elevated antibody titre may well be both a marker of a possible chronic infection, and a sign of failure of the defence mechanisms against an intracellular pathogen. It has been suggested that persistently elevated serum IgG, or in some circumstances IgA, titres may be reliable markers of chronic chlamydial infection.[30] IgA antibodies are also measurable in local secretions (e.g. in patients with chronic respiratory diseases) and their presence may help pinpoint the site of a chronic *C. pneumoniae* infection (L von Hertzen, unpublished data).

Polymerase chain reaction techniques

Polymerase chain reaction (PCR) methodology can be used to detect minute amounts of *C. pneumoniae* DNA, although a positive test does not necessarily indicate that viable organisms are present. The sensitivity of PCR investigation of respiratory secretions has been reported to be 75% as compared to serology in acute *C. pneumoniae* infection,[53] and 76.5% compared to culture and/or direct antigen detection among symptomatic and asymptomatic adults with suspected *C. pneumoniae* infections.[54] The specificity of the test has been as high as 99–100% in some studies.[54]

The low sensitivity of the PCR test in *C. pneumoniae* infections may be due to use of inappropriate sample types to detect deep-sited infections or due to the presence of inhibitors within the samples, that prevent gene amplification.[55] Specific difficulties arise with suspected chronic infections: chlamydial forms adapted to a long-term parasitic relationship with host cells have limited metabolic activity and may be undetectable by methods developed for normally growing forms.[42]

Antibiotic treatment of *C. pneumoniae* infection

As with other chlamydial species, macrolide antibiotics and tetracycline are considered appropriate first-line treatment for *C. pneumoniae* infections. The new-generation macrolides, including clarithromycin and azithromycin have high *in vitro* activity against the organism, with extensive tissue and intracellular penetration, and better tolerability than other anti-chlamydial agents (such as tetracycline).[56] The particular properties of azithromycin will be discussed elsewhere (see Chapter 6).

Grayston *et al.* found that the clinical response of *C. pneumoniae* respiratory infection to antibiotics was often slow, with persistence of symptoms and frequent clinical relapse requiring further treatment.[7] Eradicating the organism from the respiratory tract may be difficult. For example, Hammerschlag *et al.* showed, that despite treatment with tetracycline (for 2–3-weeks), 3 of 9 patients with *C. pneumoniae* respiratory illness continued to have positive cultures for the organism over an 11-month period.[57] Persistent organisms might act as a reservoir for spread of infection and could play a part in the pathogenesis of chronic disease associated with *C. pneumoniae*.

Chronic *C. pneumoniae* infections (in which the organism may alter its antigenic characteristics) may be less susceptible to eradication by antimicrobials, but data confirming this are lacking. Long-term intervention studies are also lacking and, so far, no consensus exists on the optimal treatment of chronic infection. Specific antibiotic treatment may suppress the antibody response, and this may be an important factor when using serological tests to study the exact role of this organism in various disease states.[58] However, the effect of therapy on serological markers (if any) has not been established.[59]

Summary

Chlamydia pneumoniae is one of the most common causes of infections worldwide. Most acute infections primarily involve the respiratory tract but tend to be mild or subclinical. However, the organism is also a common cause of community-acquired pneumonia. It is an obligate intracellular pathogen capable of causing latent and chronic disease and there is evidence to suggest it has a role in the pathogenesis of several inflammatory conditions. Of particular clinical relevance is the intriguing association between *C. pneumoniae* and vascular diseases. The evidence for this link is discussed in the next chapter.

References

1. Cook PJ, Honeybourne D. *Chlamydia pneumoniae. J Antimicrob Chemother* 1994; **34**: 859–73.
2. Fukusi H, Hirai K. *Chlamydia pecorum* – the 4th species of genus *Chlamydia. Microbiol Immunol* 1993; **27**: 515–22.
3. Schachter J, Caldwell HD. Chlamydiae. *Ann Rev Microbiol* 1980; **34**: 285–309.
4. Thylefors B. Present challenges in the global prevention of blindness. *Aust N Z J Ophthalmol* 1992; **20**: 89–94.
5. Witkin SS, Ledger WS. Antibody to *Chlamydia trachomatis* in sera of women with recurrent spontaneous abortions. *Am J Obs Gynecol* 1992; **167**: 135–9.
6. Schachter J, Lun L, Gooding CA, Ostler B. Pneumonitis following inclusion blennorrhoea. *J Pediatr* 1975; **87**: 779–80.
7. Grayston JT, Kuo CC, Wang SP, Altman J. A new Chlamydia psittaci strain, TWAR, isolated in acute respiratory tract infections. *N Engl J Med* 1986; **315**: 161–8.
8. Allegra L. History of a new agent of pneumonia. In: *Chlamydia pneumoniae Infection* (Allegra L, Blasi F, eds). Springer-Verlag, Milan, Italy 1995; pp.1–2.
9. Saikku P, Wang SP, Kleemola M *et al.* An epidemic of mild pneumonia due to an unusual strain of *Chlamydia psittaci. J Infect Dis* 1985; **151**: 832–9.
10. Moulder JM. Interaction of chlamydiae and host cells *in vitro. Microbiol Rev* 1991; **55**: 143–9.
11. Nurminen M, Rietschel ET, Brade H. Chemical characterisation of *Chlamydia trachomatis* lipopolysaccharide. *Infect Immun* 1985; **54**: 568–74.
12. Brade H, Brade L, Nano FE. Chemical and serological investigations on the genus-specific lipopolysaccharide epitope of *Chlamydia. Proc Natl Acad Sci USA* 1987; **84**: 2508–12.
13. Su H, Watkins NG, Zhang YX, Caldwell HD. *Chlamydia trachomatis*–host cell interactions: role of the chlamydial major outer membrane protein as an adhesin. *Infect Immun* 1990; **58**: 1017–25.
14. Brade L, Schramek S, Schade U, Brade H. Chemical, biological and immunochemical properties of *Chlamydia psittaci* lipopolysaccharide. *Infect Immun* 1986; **54**: 568–74.
15. Ingalls RR, Rice PA, Qureshi N *et al.* The inflammatory cytokine reponse to *Chlamydia trachomatis* infection is endotoxin mediated. *Infect Immun* 1995; **63**: 3125–30.
16. Schachter J. Chlamydiae. In: *Manual of Clinical Microbiology* (Balows A, Hausler W Jr, Herrmann K, Isenberg H, Shadomy J, eds). American Society of Microbiology, Washington DC, USA, 1991; pp. 1045–53.
17. Byrne GI. Host cell relationships. In: *Microbiology of Chlamydia* (Barron AL, ed.). CRC Press Inc., Florida, 1988; pp. 135–49.
18. Ward M. The immunobiology and immunopathology of *Chlamydia* infections. *APMIS* 1995; **103**: 769–96.
19. Morrison RP. Chlamydial hsp60 and the immunopathogenesis of chlamydial disease. *Semin Immunol* 1989; **3**: 25–33.
20. Grayston JT, Woolridge RL, Wang SP. Trachoma vaccine studies on Taiwan. *Ann N Y Acad Sci* 1962; **98**: 352–67.
21. Morrison RP. Chlamydial 57-kilodalton stress response protein is deleterious immune target. In: *Microbial Determinants, Virulence and Host Response* (Ayoub EM, Cassell G, Branche WC, Henry TJ, eds). Washington DC, USA, American Society of Microbiology, 1990; pp. 243–50.
22. Lindquist S, Craig EA. The heat shock proteins. *Ann Rev Genet* 1988; **22**: 631–77.
23. Young D, Lathigra R, Hendrix R, Sweetser R, Young RA. Stress proteins are immune targets in leprosy and tuberculosis. *Proc Natl Acad Sci USA* 1988; **85**: 4267–70.
24. Cerrone MC, Ma JJ, Stephens RS. Cloning and sequence of the gene for heat shock protein 60 from *Chlamydia trachomatis* and immunological reactivity of the protein. *Infect Immun* 1991; **58**: 2098–114.

25. Leinonen M. Pathogenetic mechanisms and epidemiology of *Chlamydia pneumoniae*. *Eur Heart J* 1993; **14** (Suppl. K): 57–61.
26. Grayston JT, Wang SP, Kuo CC, Campbell LA. Current knowledge on *Chlamydia pneumoniae*, strain TWAR, an important cause of pneumonia and other acute respiratory diseases. *Eur J Clin Microbiol Infect Dis* 1989; **8**: 191–202.
27. Marrie TJ, Grayston JT, Wang SP, Kno CC. Pneumonia associated with the TWAR strain of *Chlamydia*. *Ann Intern Med* 1987; **106**: 507–11.
28. Kauppinen MT, Herva E, Kujula P *et al.* The etiology of community-acquired pneumonia among hospitalized patients during a *Chlamydia pneumoniae* epidemic in Finland. *J Infect Dis* 1995; **172**: 1330–5.
29. Grayston JT, Campbell LA, Kuo CC *et al.* A new respiratory tract pathogen: *Chlamydia pneumoniae* strain TWAR. *J Infect Dis* 1990; **161**: 618–25.
30. Saikku P. The epidemiology and significance of *Chlamydia pneumoniae*. *J Infect* 1992; **1**: 27–34.
31. Ekman M-R, Grayston JT, Visakorpi R *et al.* An epidemic of infections due to *Chlamydia pneumoniae* in military conscripts. *Clin Infect Dis* 1993; **17**: 420–5.
32. Aldous MB, Grayston JT, Wang SP, Fog HM. Seroepidemiology of *Chlamydia pneumoniae* TWAR infection in Seattle families, 1966–1979. *J Infect Dis* 1992; **166**: 646–9.
33. Wang SP, Grayston JT. Population prevalence antibody to *Chlamydia pneumoniae*, strain TWAR. In: *Proceedings of the 7th International Symposium on Human Chlamydial Infections* (Bowie WR, Caldwell HD, Jones RP *et al.*, eds). 1990; pp. 402–5.
34. Kuo CC, Jackson LA, Campbell LA, Grayston JT. *Chlamydia pneumoniae* (TWAR). *Clin Microbiol Rev* 1995; **8**: 451–61.
35. Gronhagen-Riska C, Saikku P, Riska H, Froseth B, Grayston JT. Antibodies to TWAR – a novel type of Chlamydia – in sarcoidosis. In: *Sarcoidosis and Other Granulomatous Disorders* (Grassi C, Rizzato G, Pozzi E, eds). Amsterdam, Netherlands, Elsevier Science Publishers, 1988; pp. 297–301.
36. Braun J, Laitko S, Treharne J *et al. Chlamydia pneumoniae* – a new causative agent of reactive arthritis and undifferentiated oligoarthritis. *Ann Rheum Dis* 1994; **53**: 100–5.
37. Haidl S, Ivarsson S, Bjerre I, Personn K. Guillain–Barré syndrome after *Chlamydia pneumoniae* infection. *N Engl J Med* 1992; **326**: 576–7 [letter].
38. Hahn DL, Anttila T, Saikku P. Association of *Chlamydia pneumoniae* IgA antibodies with recently symptomatic asthma. *Epidemiol Infect* 1996; **117**: 513–7.
39. Beaty CD, Grayston JT, Wang SP *et al. Chlamydia pneumoniae*, strain TWAR, infection in patients with chronic obstructive pulmonary disease. *Am Rev Respir Dis* 1991; **144**: 1408-10.
40. Bone RC. *Chlamydia pneumoniae* and asthma: a potentially important relationship. *JAMA* 1991; **266**: 225–30.
41. Patton DL, Taylor HR. The histopathology of experimental trachoma: Ultrastructural changes in the conjunctival epithelium. *J Infect Dis* 1986; **153**: 870–8.
42. Beatty WL, Byrne GI, Morrison RP. Repeated and persistent infection with *Chlamydia* and the development of chronic inflammation and disease. *Trends Microbiol* 1994; **2**: 94–8.
43. Ridgway GL, Taylor-Robinson D. Current problems in microbiology: 1. Chlamydial infections: Which laboratory test? *J Clin Pathol* 1991; **44**: 1–5.
44. Schacter J, Moncada J, Dawson CR *et al.* Nonculture methods for diagnosing chlamydial infection in patients with trachoma: A clue to the pathogenesis of the disease? *J Infect Dis* 1988; **158**: 1347–52.
45. Stephens RS, Wagar EA, Edman U. Developmental regulation of tandem promoters for the major outer membrane protein gene for *Chlamydia trachomatis*. *J Bacteriol* 1988; **168**: 1277–82.

46. Puolakkainen M, Parker J, Kuo CC, Grayston JT, Campbell LA. Characterisation of a *Chlamydia pneumoniae* epitope recognised by species-specific monoclonal antibodies. In: *Proceedings of 8th International Symposium on Human Chlamydial Infections*, (Orfila J, Byrne GI, Chernesky MA *et al.*, eds). Bologna, Italy, Societa Editrice Esculapoi, 1994; pp. 185–8.
47. Wang SP, Grayston JT. Microimmunofluorescence antibody responses in *Chlamydia trachomatis* infection, a review. In: *Chlamydial Infections* (Mårdh PA *et al.*, eds). Amsterdam, Netherlands, Elseiver Biomed Press, 1970; pp. 301–16.
48. Grayston JT, Golubjatnikov R, Hagiwara T *et al.* Serologic tests for *Chlamydia pneumoniae*. *Pediatr Infect Dis J* 1993; **12**: 790–1.
49. Peeling RW, Wang SP, Grayston JT *et al.* Chlamydia serology: Inter-laboratory variation in microimmunofluorescence results. *Proceedings from the 9th International Symposium on Human Chlamydial Infection*, Napa, California USA (June 21–26, 1998).
50. Brade L, Brunnemann H, Ernst M *et al.* Occurrence of antibodies against chlamydial lipopolysaccharide in human sera as measured by ELISA using an artificial glycoconjugate antigen. *FEMS Immunol Med Microbiol* 1994; **8**: 27–41.
51. Verkooyen RP, Van Lent NA, Mousavi SA *et al.* Diagnosis of *Chlamydia pneumoniae* in patients with chronic obstructive pulmonary disease by microimmunofluorescence and ELISA. *J Med Microbiol* 1997; **46**: 959–64.
52. Wang SP and Grayston JT. Microimmunofluorescence serological studies with the TWAR organism. In: *Chlamydial Infections* (Oriel JD, Ridgway G, Schachter J, *et al.*, eds). Cambridge, UK, Cambridge University Press, 1986; pp. 329–32.
53. Thom DH, Grayston JT, Campbell LA *et al.* Respiratory infection with *Chlamydia pneumoniae* in middle-aged and older adult outpatients. *Eur J Clin Microbiol Infect Dis* 1994; **13**: 785–92.
54. Gaydos CA, Roblin PM, Hammerschlag MR *et al.* Diagnostic utility of PCR-enzyme immunoassay, culture, and serology for detection of *Chlamydia pneumoniae* in symptomatic and asymptomatic patients. *J Clin Microbiol* 1994; **32**: 903–5.
55. Soini H, Shurnik M, Liippo K, Tala E, Viljanen MK. Detection and identification of mycobacteria by amplification of a segment of the gene coding for the 32-kilodalton protein. *J Clin Microbiol* 1992; **30**: 2025–8.
56. Williams JD. The new azalide antimicrobials. *Curr Opin Infect Dis* 1994; **7**: 653–7.
57. Hammerschlag MR, Chirgwin K, Roblin PM *et al.* Persistent infection with *Chlamydia pneumoniae* following acute respiratory illness. *Clin Infect Dis* 1992; **14**: 178–82.
58. Bourke SJ, Lightfoot NF. *Chlamydia pneumoniae*: Defining the clinical spectrum of infection requires precise laboratory diagnosis. *Thorax* 1995; **50** (Suppl 1): S43–8.
59. Grayston JT. Antibiotic treatment of *Chlamydia pneumoniae* for secondary prevention of cardiovascular events. *Circulation* 1998; **97**: 1669–70.

Chapter 4: Association of *Chlamydia pneumoniae* with atherosclerosis: The evidence

Introduction

An association between chlamydial infection and vascular disease was first described about 60 years ago. In the 1940s, South America investigators observed that the intradermal Frei test (which measures hypersensitivity to all chlamydial species) was positive not only in patients with lymphogranuloma venerum, but often also in patients with arteriosclerosis.[1] At the time, these observations went largely unacknowledged, possibly because they were published only in Spanish. It is now clear that all chlamydial species can cause endocarditis, myocarditis or pericarditis.[2] In addition, evidence accumulated since the late 1980s from seroepidemiological, pathological and animal studies suggests that *Chlamydia pneumoniae* may have a direct role in the development or progression of atherosclerosis and, in particular, coronary heart disease (CHD).

Seroepidemiological studies

Links with CHD

Early observations

Saikku *et al.* were the first group to describe an apparent association between *C. pneumoniae* and CHD, in 1988.[3] These investigators conducted a case–control study in which 26 of 38 (68%) consecutive males presenting with acute myocardial infarction (MI) had a raised titre of antibodies against an epitope of chlamydial lipopolysaccharide (LPS), a raised titre was present in only 3% of a control group and absent in patients with chronic CHD. Furthermore, IgG and IgA anti-*C. pneumoniae* antibody titres (measured using an microimmunofluorescence assay) were, in general, elevated significantly in the cardiac patients (i.e. those with chronic CHD or acute MI) compared with titres in the controls. The investigators suggested that acute MI might be associated with an exacerbation of underlying chronic *C. pneumoniae* infection: in these patients, seroconversion might be a sign of a sudden imbalance between the relative amounts of chlamydial LPS and of antibodies directed against this antigen. The study was limited by the absence of a prospective design and the fact that there was no controlling for smoking and other cardiovascular risk factors.

Further retrospective data

Since the first case–control study, the association between elevated anti-*C. pneumoniae* antibody titres and atherosclerosis has been verified in 22 seroepidemiological studies performed worldwide over the last decade. Some of the principal studies are discussed below.

In Seattle, USA, Thom *et al.* showed that, compared with controls (i.e. people with normal coronary arteries), patients with angiographically diagnosed CHD had greater mean anti-*C. pneumoniae* antibody levels:[4] those with IgG antibody titres of 1/64 or greater were twice as likely as those with lower titres to have atherosclerotic lesions. However, these results were not stastistically significant, and the study did not control for smoking. In a further study conducted by the same investigators, 171 cases were compared to 120 matched controls. Patients undergoing coronary angiography who had an elevated IgG titre (≥1/8) against *C. pneumoniae* were around twice as likely as those without raised titres to have angiographically detectable CHD (odds ratio 2.6 [1.4–4.8]).[5] These differences persisted even after adjustments for certain cardiovascular risk factors (including serum cholesterol concentration, hypertension, diabetes mellitus and social class). However, it appeared that the association between raised anti-*C. pneumoniae* antibody titre and CHD was confined to smokers (an odds ratio of 3.5 for ever-smokers versus 0.8 for lifelong non-smokers). Furthermore, the association was weaker (odds ratio 1.2) when subjects with normal coronary angiograms rather than members of the general population were used as controls. The authors concluded that the results of their study provided some (but not conclusive) evidence of an association between *C. pneumoniae* seropositivity and CHD.

Work based at a UK institution has shown an association between seropositivity to *C. pneumoniae* and prevalent CHD in a community cross-sectional survey,[6] so corroborating the original findings of Finnish and American investigators.[3,5] In particular, the study demonstrated a strong correlation between the presence of an elevated serum anti-*C. pneumoniae* IgG titre (≥1/64) and CHD (odds ratio about 7), that was independent of age, social class and conventional cardiovascular risk factors (see Table 6). In the same study, a comparison was made between the antibody titres of a group of 100 males (age 45–65 years) with angiographically demonstrable CHD and those of a matched control group (without angina and with normal electrocardiographs, n=64). Both anti-*C. pneumoniae* IgA and IgG subclasses of antibodies were elevated significantly in the CHD group. An extension of this investigation assessed the relationship between *C. pneumoniac* seropositivity and certain serum cardiovascular risk factors.[7] Elevated serum fibrinogen, factor VIIa and CRP levels were found to be associated with a raised anti-*C. pneumoniae* antibody titre, suggesting that any harmful effects of infection in atherosclerosis may be mediated by activation of inflammatory and procoagulant markers.

Table 6: Effect of adjustment for various cardiovascular risk factors on the relationship between anti-*C. pneumoniae* (Cp) antibody titre (IgG) and CHD

Odds ratios – titres adjusted for	**All Cp titres (16+)**	**Low Cp titres (16–32)**	**High Cp (64+)**
Nothing	2.2*	1.6	7.3**
Age alone	2.0*	1.5	6.6**
Age and risk factors	2.0	1.5	6.9**
Age, risk factors and social class	1.9	1.5	6.1*

*$p<0.05$; **$p<0.01$ (Adapted from Mendall MA, Carrington D, Strachan DP *et al.* *Chlamydia pneumoniae*: risk factors for serpositivity and association with coronary heart disease. *J Infect* 1995; **30**: 121–8, with permission.)

In three other studies, (one based in the UK,[8] the other two in Italy[9,10]) a significant proportion of patients admitted with acute MI or unstable angina had serological evidence of chronic or previous *C. pneumoniae* infection. These results provide further circumstantial evidence of an association between serological markers of this infection and acute coronary events.

Immune complex studies

Chlamydia pneumoniae immune complexes have been found in about 60% of the patients with acute MI.[11] During convalescence from the acute event, the immune complex pattern appears to shift from chlamydial antigen excess to anti-chlamydial antibody excess. The presence of immune complexes containing bacterial proteins suggests that there may be a chronic *C. pneumoniae* infection very close to the lumen of blood vessels and that the organism's components are shed directly into the circulation.[12]

Prospective data

Additional evidence suggesting that *C. pneumoniae* might be involved in the pathogenesis of atherosclerosis was provided by a nested case–control study of sera collected prospectively from the Helsinki Heart Study.[13] These samples were used to investigate the relation between anti-*C. pneumoniae* antibody titres and subsequent development of CHD. Elevated IgA titres against *C. pneumoniae* and the presence of immune complexes containing *C. pneumoniae* LPS antigen were associated with an increased risk of developing a cardiac event 3–6 months after the sera had been collected (odds ratio 2.3, 95% confidence level [CI] 1.3–5.2). These associations were independent of age, blood pressure and smoking habit. Patients who had high IgA titres at both the beginning and the end of the study (suggesting persistent *C. pneumoniae* infection) were more likely to suffer a cardiac event during the interim. In contrast to other studies, there was no apparent evidence of a relationship between IgG anti-*C. pneumoniae* antibody titres and CHD.

A larger prospective study of subjects in two areas of Finland recorded all cardiac events during a 7-year follow-up period.[14] Elevated anti-*C. pneumoniae* antibody titres (IgG ≥1/128 and IgA ≥1/40) at baseline were associated with an increased risk of developing such events in non-diabetic subjects in eastern Finland, but not in diabetic patients in western Finland. There was no obvious explanation for the epidemiological pattern of these results.

A subsequent nested case–control study (54 cases and 108 age-matched controls) conducted in the Netherlands (during 1985–1990) showed that an elevated anti-*C. pneumoniae* antibody titres was associated with an increased independent risk of developing CHD (i.e. cardiac death, MI or angina), with odds ratio 2.8 (95% CI: 1.3–5.8).[15] Interestingly, no association was demonstrable between CHD and seropositivity to either *Helicobacter pylori* or cytomegalovirus.

Links with cerebrovascular disease

Asymptomatic disease

Elevated anti-*C. pneumoniae* antibody titres are also linked with atherosclerosis in non-cardiac arteries. For example, in a case–control study, Melnick *et al.* reported that 73% of adults with asymptomatic carotid artery thickening (as determined by ultrasonography) had serological evidence of previous *C. pneumoniae* infection (i.e. raised IgG antibody levels), compared with 63% of controls matched by age, gender, ethnicity, time of recruitment and study centre.[16] There remained a twofold higher prevalence of carotid atherosclerosis in those with elevated anti-*C. pneumoniae* antibody titres even after adjustment for differences in blood pressure, prevalence of diabetes mellitus, cigarette smoking habit, serum low-density-lipoprotein (LDL)-cholesterol concentration and level of education. The odds ratio for the association between raised titres and atherosclerosis was higher in younger patients (those aged 45–54 years) than that for those aged 55–64 years (odds ratio 3.5 versus 1.59).

Clinically overt disease

Wimmer *et al.* investigated anti-*C. pneumoniae* antibody titres in 58 consecutive patients with recent cerebrovascular disease (stroke or transient ischaemic event) and 52 controls (matched for, age, gender and locality).[17] Patients with a recent cerebrovascular event were more likely than the controls to have a positive IgA anti-*C. pneumoniae* antibody titre and evidence of *C. pneumoniae*-containing immune complexes (odds ratio 2), even after adjusting for age, gender, hypertension and history of migraine. This finding was corroborated by investigators in another study who showed that serological markers of both acute and chronic *C. pneumoniae* infection were significantly more prevalent in patients with strokes and transient cerebral ischaemia (n=176), than in matched hospital controls (n=1518).[18] There were no differences between haemorrhagic or infarction-related strokes with regard to the relationship with the serum markers nor was there any association between anti-*C. pneumoniae* seropositivity and serum lipid or fibrinogen concentration.

Does smoking confound the seroepidemiological data?

Cigarette smoking renders individuals susceptible to respiratory infections and atherosclerotic diseases and could, therefore, be an important confounder in any link between *C. pneumoniae* and vascular disease. In support of this suggestion, an investigation of 365 patients with respiratory disease conducted by Hahn and Golubjatnikov showed a small, but significant, association between smoking and seroconversion to *C. pneumoniae*.[19] Individuals in this study were younger (mean age 34 years) than in most other clinical studies on *C. pneumoniae* and CHD. In addition, all the patients studied had a current respiratory illness (whereas random or healthy controls were used in most other studies). Karvonen *et al.* assessed the relationship between smoking and *C. pneumoniae* seropositivity in a larger cohort of subjects (n=2346).[20] Overall, the prevalence of *C. pneumoniae* IgG seropositivity was 50% higher among 'ever-smokers' than among non-smokers. Seropositivity was also higher among males and younger patients.

Most other studies have, however, shown that even after controlling for cigarette smoking (and other traditional risk factors), anti-*C. pneumoniae* antibody titre remains an independent risk factor for having evidence of CHD.[6,13] Even if smoking does expose the individual to chronic *C. pneumoniae* infection, this does not exclude the possibility that the microorganism is involved in the pathogenesis of atherosclerosis. It could even be that some of the harmful effects of cigarette smoking on the vasculature rely on the presence of chronic *C. pneumoniae* infection.

Negative studies

In contrast to many studies demonstrating a positive link between anti-*C. pneumoniae* antibodies and CHD, a few have shown no such association.

A case–control epidemiological study conducted in Israel demonstrated no significant difference in the prevalence of anti-*C. pneumoniae* seropositivity (anti-IgA or anti-IgG antibodies) in 302 patients with acute MI and 486 age- and sex-matched population controls.[21] (The investigators did, however, acknowledge that a possible recent outbreak of community-acquired *C. pneumoniae* infection could have obscured any association between *C. pneumoniae* and CHD.) Similarly, Weiss *et al.* could demonstrate no correlation between IgG anti-*C. pneumoniae* antibody titres and CHD: no difference was found between antibody titres in a group of patients undergoing coronary atherectomy procedures (n=65) compared with asymptomatic controls (n=28).[22] Finally, in a preliminary report, Altman *et al.* presented evidence, that a raised anti-*C. pneumoniae* antibody titre was not an independent predictor of further non-fatal vascular events in 159 patients with severe arterial disease.[23] However, the control group in this study comprised 203 patients with heart valve prostheses (but no arterial disease) rather than a conventional control group made up of subjects without evidence of cardiac disease.

Strengths and limitations of serological data

A review of the evidence linking the presence of anti-*C. pneumoniae* antibodies with and that of CHD found that most of the relevant studies found odds ratios of at least 2 or higher in favour of such an association (see Figure 6).[24] Indeed, some studies reported that odds ratios increased with the antibody titre. The studies were performed in various populations with different criteria being used to define cases and to adjust for potential confounders. In addition, some of the serological studies can be criticised with regards to the anti-*C. pneumoniae* titre cut-offs arbitrarily selected to indicate seropositivity, the types of controls used and the borderline statistical significances of many of the study results. Whether an elevated antibody titre is a reliable indicator of underlying *C. pneumoniae* infection, or simply a reflection of antigenic cross-reactivity, is also unclear.[25] Establishing the existence of a causal association between such *C. pneumoniae* infection and CHD is also hampered by the wide variation in antibody responses to the organism, attributable to differences in the mode of infection or the original infective dose or any previous exposure.

Despite these factors, findings have generally been consistent from study to study, suggesting the existence of a true association between *C. pneumoniae* and CHD.

Direct examination of atheromatous plaques

In addition to seroepidemiological data, evidence for an association between *C. pneumoniae* and atherosclerosis has come from tissue examination of arterial plaque material (see Table 7).

Figure 6: Epidemiological studies of *C. pneumoniae* seropositivity and atherosclerotic disease

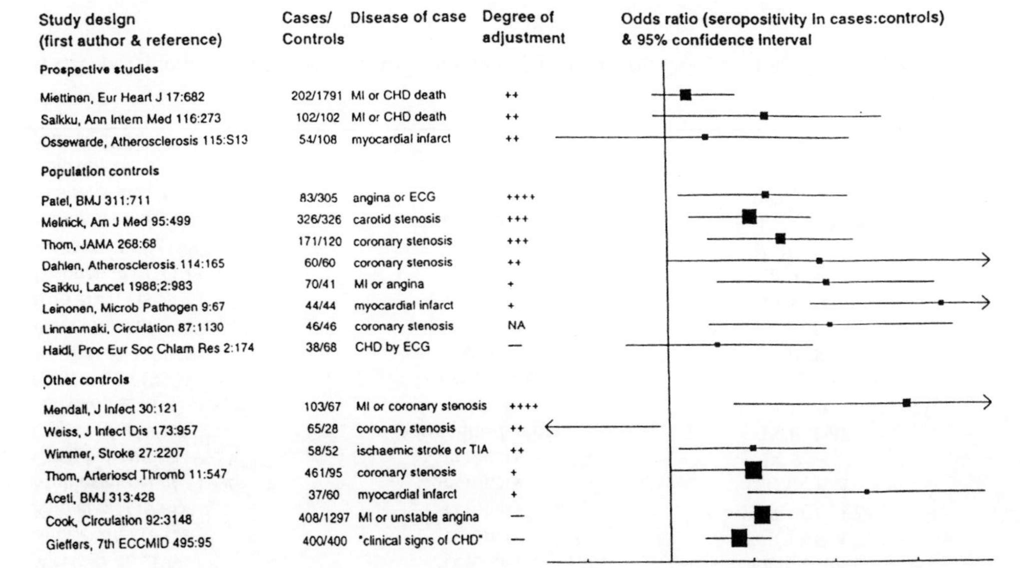

NA = no adjustments were made, although measurements were made for confounders; TIA = transient ischaemic attack. Other abbreviations and definitions as in Figure 3. (Adapted from Danesh J, Collins R, Peto R. Chronic infections and coronary heart disease: Is there a link? *Lancet* 1997; **350**: 430–6, with permission.)

Table 7: Key published studies examining for the presence of *C. pneumoniae* in atherosclerotic specimens

Reference	Atherosclerotic specimen	Method of detection	Proportion of positive specimens
Weiss *et al.* (1996)[22]	coronary	PCR, culture	1/56, 0/22
Shor *et al.* (1992)[26]	coronary	ICC, EM	5/7, 7/7
Kuo *et al.* (1993)[27]	coronary	PCR, ICC, EM	13/30, 15/36, 6/21
Muhlestein *et al.* (1996)[29]	coronary	IMF, EM	71/90, 3/5
Campbell *et al.* (1995)[30]	coronary	PCR, ICC	12/38, 17/38
Ong *et al.* (1996)[31]	aorta, illio-femoral	PCR, IMF	15/35, 3/12
Grayston *et al.* (1995)[32]	carotid	PCR, ICC	3/5, 36/61
Chiu *et al.* (1997)[33]	carotid, aorta	ICC	54/76
Blasi *et al.* (1996)[34]	aorta	PCR	26/51
Paterson *et al.* (1998)[38]	coronary, carotid	PCR	0/30
Kuo *et al.* (1995)[39]	coronary	PCR, ICC	3/18, 7/18
Juvonen *et al.* (1997)[40]	aorta	PCR, ICC, EM	6/6, 12/12, 3/4
Jackson *et al.* (1997)[42]	carotid	PCR, ICC, culture	6/25, 8/16 1/25
Ramirez *et al.* (1996)[43]	coronary	PCR, ICC, EM, culture	3/10, 5/10, 3/10, 1/10
Maass *et al.* (1998)[45]	coronary	PCR, culture	21/70, 11/70
Tuazon, 1996[70]	coronary	PCR	4/40
Maass, 1997[71]	carotid	PCR	9/61

(PCR=polymerase chain reaction, ICC=immunocytochemistry, EM=electron microscopy, IMF= immunofluorescence)

Coronary arteries at autopsy

The presence of *C. pneumoniae* in atherosclerotic lesions was first reported by Shor *et al.* in South Africa.[26] These investigators examined autopsy coronary artery sections from patients dying of trauma. They demonstrated 'chlamydia-like' structures in seven out of seven specimens using electron microscopy; five of these samples were also positive by immunocytochemical staining for *C. pneumoniae.* An expanded study of autopsy cases (aged 20–83 years) also from South Africa, undertaken in collaboration with investigators in Seattle, USA, tested coronary plaque lesions for *C. pneumoniae* using both polymerase chain reaction (PCR) techniques and immunohistochemical analysis.[27] Of 36 subjects dying from non-cardiac causes, the organism was detected in 20 (56%) using one or both methods. In six of 21 lesions, the typical pear-shaped *C. pneumoniae* organisms were demonstrable by electron microscopy (see Figure 7). *Chlamydia pneumoniae* was found only within sites of tissue damage, including the lipid-rich core of atheromatous plaques, smooth muscle cells and necrotic areas of the plaque; no organisms were detected in normal tissue adjacent to the sclerotic lesions nor in normal coronary arteries from 11 control patients. Post-humous testing (using microimmunofluorescence techniques) of sera from 34 of the positive cases (i.e. patients with *C. pneumoniae* in autopsy plaque specimens) revealed that 26 had significantly raised IgG anti-*C. pneumoniae* antibody titres. Intriguingly, the organsim was also detected in plaques from six of eight antibody-negative cases, 14 of 20 with a low antibody titre (1/8–1/32) and none of six with high titre (1/64–1/512). This lack of correlation between demonstrable *C. pneumoniae* organisms in tissue samples and antibody seropositivity has raised questions about the interpretation of sero-epidemiological data apparently linking *C. pneumoniae* and CHD. A possible explanation of these findings is that organisms lodged deep within well-developed atheromatous lesions might not continuously stimulate antibody production or, at least, antibody levels detectable by microimmunofluorescence.

These doubts are challenged by the work of Davidson *et al.*[28] These investigators tested for the presence of *C. pneumoniae* within autopsy coronary artery specimens from 60 indigenous Alaskan natives (at low risk of CHD; mean age of 34.1 years) who had died primarily from non-cardiovascular causes, and compared such findings with titres of anti-*C. pneumoniae* antibodies, from sera from the same subjects drawn from a mean of 8.8 years before death. The coronary artery specimens were examined histologically and graded for atherosclerotic changes, and checked for the presence of *C. pneumoniae* using PCR and immunocytochemical techniques. Serological markers of infection were assessed using a microimmunofluorescence assay. *Chlamydia pneumoniae* was demonstrated positive by PCR or immunocytochemical staining in the coronary arteries of 22 of 60 (37%) subjects. The organism was frequently found within macrophage foam cells, and in specimens with raised fibrolipid plaques. Interestingly, the odds ratio for the presence of *C. pneumoniae* within a raised atheromatous plaque in patients with an IgG antibody ≥1/256 more than 8 years earlier was 6.1 (95%CI 1.1–36.6), and for all coronary artery specimens after adjustment for confounding variables, 9.4 (95%CI 2.6–33.8). The study provided the first evidence that infection with *C. pneumoniae* may precede or accompany early asymptomatic atheromatous lesions that harbour the intracellular pathogen in young adults. It has also been suggested there may be a 'dose-response' criterion of causality – with regard to both the grade of the atherosclerotic lesion and the height of anti-*C. pneumoniae* antibody titre: accordingly, greater serum levels of anti-*C. pneumoniae* antibody titres in CHD may prove to be a clearer indicator of the presence of endovascular infection. Further investigations are needed to help confirm and define the temporal sequence of events with regard to chronic *C. pneumoniae* infection, its potential interactions with conventional cardiovascular risk factors and the development of atherosclerosis.

In vivo examination of coronary artherectomy samples

Muhlestein *et al.* tested for the presence of *Chlamydia* species using direct immunofluorescence in plaque specimens from 90 patients undergoing coronary atherectomy for symptomatic angina.[29] Twenty-four autopsy control specimens from patients without atherosclerosis were also examined. A markedly higher proportion of the atheromatous tissue specimens from the patients with CHD were positive for

Chlamydia species when compared with those from controls (79% versus 4%; $p<0.001$). Transmission electron microscopy confirmed the presence of the organism in three of five positive specimens. Although the presence of a primary non-restenotic lesion predicted the presence of *Chlamydia*, clinical factors did not.

Chlamydia pneumoniae has also been demonstrated in atherectomy specimens from patients with angina[30] and in atheromatous arteries of patients with other vascular diseases.[31–33] For example, *C. pneumoniae* DNA was detected in aortic plaque tissue from 26 of 51 patients undergoing abdominal aortic aneurysm surgery.[34] Nearly 90% (23 of 26) of the positive cases had serological evidence of past *C. pneumoniae* infection, two had an acute 'reinfection pattern' and only one was seronegative. By contrast, only nine of 25 patients with plaques negative for *C. pneumoniae* on PCR testing had serology consistent with chronic *C. pneumoniae* infection ($p<0.01$). Juvonen *et al.* have corroborated these findings and found evidence of chlamydial LPS and antigens in abdominal aortic aneurysms but not in control samples from healthy aortic tissue.[35]

Figure 7: Transmission electron micrograph of endosomes in foam cell with elementary bodies of *C. pneumoniae*

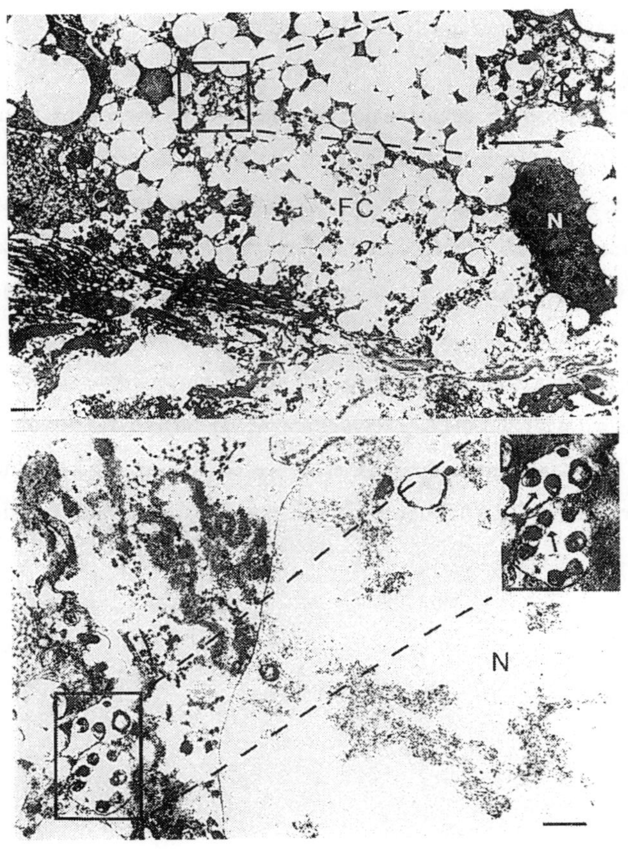

Bar = 0.5μm; N = nucleus, FC = foam cell. Arrows in inset point to elementary bodies. (Reproduced from Kuo CC, Shor A, Campbell LA *et al*. Demonstration of *Chlamydia pneumoniae* in atherosclerotic lesions of coronary arteries. *J Infect Dis* 1993; **167**: 841–9, with permission of University of Chicago Press.)

Meta-analysis data and potential implications of plaque studies

Since the original observations reported in 1992,[26] over 20 published studies have now found evidence of *C. pneumoniae* organisms in atherosclerotic vessels. By contrast, the organism has been identified only rarely in 'healthy' control arteries.[31,36]

In a meta-analysis of 13 studies that sought *C. pneumoniae* in human pathology samples,[24] evidence of the organism within endovascular tissue (defined by the presence of chlamydial DNA, antigens or elementary bodies) was found in 52% (257 of 495) of atheromatous lesions. This compared with only 5% (6 of 118) of control non-atheromatous arteries (odds ratio 10 [95% CI 5–22]). The difficulty in finding arterial samples that are completely atheroma-free in older individuals has meant few of these studies have sampled tissue from age- and gender-matched controls. Nevertheless, only a minority of studies have not found any evidence of *C. pneumoniae* in atherosclerotic vessels.[22,37,38] The organism has even been found in early arterial lesions in teenagers.[39]

The findings of the plaque studies (in tandem with the seroepidemiological data) provide strong circumstantial evidence that *C. pneumoniae* could be involved in the pathogenesis of atherosclerosis. However, since *C. pneumoniae* is a ubiquitous organism and has been identified in non-vascular, non-respiratory sites (such as stenosed aortic valves,[40] hepatic vessels[31] and spleen[41]) it has been suggested that it is merely an 'innocent bystander' in inflamed arterial tissue. Somewhat against this idea, however, a recent autopsy study has shown a higher prevalence of *C. pneumoniae*-positive samples in the cardiovascular tissue of patients who had died of CHD than in patients who had died of non-cardiac causes (64% versus 38%).[42]

Culture of *C. pneumoniae* from atheroma

Chlamydia pneumoniae organisms have been successfully isolated from atheromatous vessels and then cultured *in vitro*. A single viable strain of *C. pneumoniae* was isolated from a diseased coronary artery of one patient undergoing cardiac transplantation[43] and from a carotid endarterectomy specimen taken from another.[44] The rarity of such isolation in comparison to the much higher rates of detection of *C. pneumoniae* antigen and DNA by immunocytochemical (ICC) and PCR techniques is similar to the position with other chronic chlamydial infections. For instance, in trachoma and pelvic inflammatory disease, *C. trachomatis* antigen or DNA may be demonstrated in a high proportion of affected tissue samples, while the viable organism itself is rarely isolated (perhaps suggesting that such organisms may persist in the host in a viable but non-replicative state).

In one study, Maass *et al.* cultured replicating *C. pneumoniae* from 11 of 70 (16%) atherosclerotic samples obtained during myocardial revascularisation (i.e. restenotic bypass segments and coronary endarterectomy samples).[45] A higher proportion of the samples (21 out of 70; 30%) were PCR-positive for *C. pneumoniae*. No positive results were obtained from 17 control samples that had no macroscopic features of atherosclerosis. Of additional interest, neither anti-*C. pneumoniae* serology nor clinical characteristics helped in identifying those patients with endovascular *C. pneumoniae* infection. Only six out of 21 patients with *C. pneumoniae* in plaque tissue also had elevated anti-*C. pneumoniae* antibody titres; by contrast, such elevated titres were seen in six patients without detectable *C. pneumoniae* organisms.

The distribution of *C. pneumoniae* in the coronary arteries is thought to be highly heterogenous: this could explain the difficulty in culturing the organism from atheromatous plaques. The small amounts of tissue samples generally available for testing and the effects of freeze–storage procedures on *C. pneumoniae* may have also hampered attempts to isolate the organism.

Nevertheless, evidence that a significant proportion of coronary arteries occluded by atheroma may harbour viable *C. pneumoniae* favours a pathogenetic role for such infection in atherogenesis and argues against a purely commensal or 'bystander' presence of replicative organisms.

Evidence from peripheral blood PCR studies

Attempts to establish whether *C. pneumoniae* has a causal role in atherosclerosis and CHD have been hampered by diagnostic difficulties. There is no doubt that the organism can be often found in blood vessels, where its exact role remains unclear. Unfortunately, no simple, reliable test is available for identifying people with vascular *C. pneumoniae* infection. And there are legitimate concerns that serological tests may be unreliable markers of chronic *C. pneumoniae* infection. For example, in some investigations, it has become clear that a chronic *C. pneumoniae* infection may occur in the absence of any related continuing antibody response. In light of these diagnostic problems, it is interesting that promising preliminary reports show that PCR techniques may offer a way of detecting *C. pneumoniae* DNA in the peripheral circulation. For instance, Naidu *et al.* were able to demonstrate such DNA in the sera of a large proportion of subjects with either acute MI or chronic CHD, and much more frequently than in sera from age- and gender-matched controls without CHD.[46] Interestingly, *C. pneumoniae* DNA positivity was most prevalent among those who had *C. pneumoniae* antibody titres of ≥1/32. These findings (which need confirmation) suggest that DNA might be liberated continuously or intermittently from degenerating *C. pneumoniae* organisms in vessels or elsewhere.

Since *C. pneumoniae* may be carried in human monocytes, these cells may provide a method of diagnosing such infection. In the comparable case of active *Mycobacterium tuberculosis* infection, Condos *et al.* showed that peripheral blood-based PCR detection was a technically feasible approach not only for diagnosing pulmonary tuberculosis infection but also for monitoring the efficacy of therapy.[47] This diagnostic approach has now been tested in patients with CHD who have presumed *C. pneumoniae* infection. Using a validated nested PCR method to detect the presence of *C. pneumoniae* DNA within peripheral monocytes, Boman *et al.* investigated 103 patients undergoing coronary angiography for suspected CHD and 52 (presumed healthy) blood donors.[48] Fifty-nine percent of the patients with CHD were PCR-positive to *C. pneumoniae*, but somewhat surprisingly, so were 46% of the (unmatched) controls. The high degree of positivity in both populations, contrasts with the much lower rates reported by Wong *et al.*[49] In their investigation, 48 of 621 (7.7%) males with CHD had monocytes positive for *C. pneumoniae* compared with only 3 of 121 (2.5%) without CHD (odds ratio (OR) 3.29 [95% CI 1.01–10.76, p=0.04]).

Further studies are attempting to refine the blood-based PCR technique, and with the aim of ultimately providing a validated means of identifying carriers of *C. pneumoniae*. Whether such a test could supersede the microimmunofluorescence assay and other serological tests remains to be seen.

Animal models

Chlamydia pneumoniae is transmitted from person to person; no animal reservoir for human infection has been identified.[50] However, chlamydial strains closely related to *C. pneumoniae* have been found in animals, and in the laboratory, contact animals have been shown to be susceptible to experimentally induced infection with *C. pneumoniae*.[51,52] The potential for an interaction between *C. pneumoniae*, the host immune system and subsequent tissue damage in chronic diseases, in particular atherosclerosis, has, therefore, been studied using animal models.

Evidence of systemic spread and persistent infection

In various studies, different monkey species (including baboons, Rhesus and cynomolgus monkeys) were infected deliberately by *C. pneumoniae* (strain TWAR) using a number of challenge routes.[53,54] No signs of clinical disease were noted post-inoculation, although *C. pneumoniae* could be recovered from the nasopharynx of the animals. In the cynomolgus monkey, the organism persisted for a prolonged period and was demonstrated in rectal swabs after intranasal inoculation, suggesting systemic spread of the microorganism had occurred.[54]

Experimental mouse models have been developed to elucidate further the natural history and immunopathogenesis of *C. pneumoniae* infection.[55–58] Finnish investigators have shown that after intranasal inoculation of such animals with *C. pneumoniae*, the microorganism can be isolated from lung tissue for more than 2 weeks after initial challenge.[56] In the mouse model of Yang *et al.*, deliberate primary infection with *C. pneumoniae* induced an acute pneumonia – with infiltration of polymorphonuclear leucocytes and exudate in lung alveoli and bronchi – followed by a monocytic infiltrate.[57] Long after initial infection, the organism may remain in a 'latent' stage and be reactivated in states of immunosuppression (e.g. following steroid treatment[59,60]). Intranasal inoculation of mice with *C. pneumoniae* has also shown that the organism can spread systemically to, for example, lymph nodes, the spleen and the lung. The most plausible method of spread is via infected macrophages.[61]

Deliberate repeated infection of New Zealand White rabbits with *C. pneumoniae* leads to respiratory disease and granuloma formation, which resembles that seen in human sarcoidosis.[15] In addition, *C. pneumoniae* may spread systemically and has been isolated by PCR from splenic tissue and peripheral blood mononuclear cells.[62]

Chlamydia pneumoniae-induced atherosclerosis

In one study, multiple intranasal inoculations of apolipoprotein E apoE-deficient mice (which spontaneously develop atherosclerosis) with *C. pneumoniae* resulted in the microorganism being subsequently detectable within atherosclerotic areas of the aortas of 15–100% of mice.[63] Subsequently, Fong *et al.* showed that six New Zealand White rabbits infected deliberately with *C. pneumoniae* developed pneumonia, and two of the animals also developed fatty streaks and grade III atherosclerotic lesions in the aorta, 1-2 weeks after infection.[64] In other experiments, Laitinen *et al.* inoculated rabbits intranasally with *C. pneumoniae*.[65] No atherosclerotic changes were detected in animals after a single infection. However, following deliberate reinfection with *C. pneumoniae*, six of nine animals developed inflammatory changes, intimal thickening and fibroid plaques resembling atherosclerosis in their aortas. Immunohistochemical tests for *C. pneumoniae* antigen were positive in all of these animals. A series of control animals had no signs of atherosclerosis.

In the largest animal study to date, New Zealand White rabbits received repeated intranasal inoculations of either *C. pneumoniae* (n=20) or saline control (n=10), at 3-week intervals, and were fed a diet supplemented with cholesterol.[66] After the final inoculation, infected and control rabbits were randomised to a 7-week course of the antibiotic azithromycin or to no therapy. At 3 months, the animals were sacrificed and sections of their aortas examined for intimal thickening and checked for the presence of *C. pneumoniae* using immunofluorescence technique. The results showed that intimal thickening was most marked in the infected animals compared with control animals (0.55 mm versus 0.16 mm; $p<0.025$) but that such changes did not occur in infected animals given azithromycin. *Chlamydia pneumoniae* antigen was detected in two untreated, and three treated animals, but was not detected in any of the control animals (see Figure 8).

Figure 8: Photomicrographs of representative aortic sections from animals in the infected/untreated group (**A**); control (uninfected/untreated) (**B**); and infected/treated (**C**). Haematoxylin and eosin-stained section, original magnification x100.

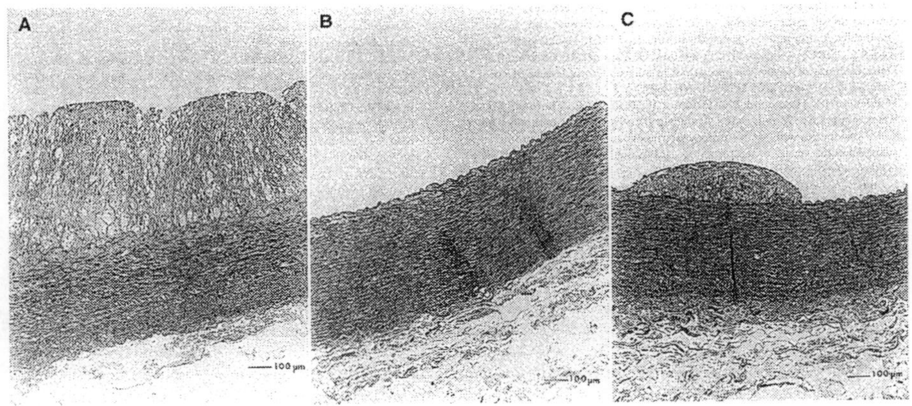

(Reproduced from Muhlestein JB, Anderson JL, Hammon EH *et al.* Infection with *Chlamydia pneumoniae* accelerates the development of atherosclerosis and treatment with azithromycin prevents it in a rabbit model. *Circulation* 1998; **97**: 633–6, with permission.)

Implications of preliminary animal model studies

The animal models reported to date, although based on small numbers, suggest that *C. pneumoniae* infection may be capable of initiating atheromatous changes,[64,65] and that azithromycin can limit the atherogenic effects of such infection.[66] The extent to which atherosclerosis has developed or been accelerated in such animals has varied, suggesting differences in the ease of establishing persistent *C. pneumoniae* infection or in the host response to such infection. Infection-related atherosclerosis in the models may occur in the absence of detectable local chlamydial antigen, and antibiotic therapy may not immediately eliminate such antigen. Furthermore, the contributory effect (if any) of a cholesterol-rich diet is unclear, the optimal antibiotic dosage to prevent atherosclerosisis is not known and, of course, animal models of atherosclerosis may not mirror human atherogenesis. Nevertheless, these early experimental animal models support the notion of a causal relationship between *C. pneumoniae* and atherogenesis.

What about Koch's postulates?

Conventionally, for an infective agent to be established as a direct cause of CHD, it would need to satisfy Koch's postulates.[67] This would mean that: the microorganism, would be present in all, or nearly all, cases of the disease; inoculations of its pure cultures would produce disease (for example, when injected into susceptible animals); the microorganism would be obtainable from these diseased states; and it could then be propagated in pure culture. So far the first – and, possibly, the second – of these postulates appear to be fulfilled with respect to *C. pneumoniae* in CHD. However, some workers have argued that Koch's postulates may lack sufficient sensitivity to be used for dismissing the possibility of a causal link between an infectious agent and a given disease.[68] Indeed, it is worth remembering that *H. pylori* does not satisfy the requirements of Koch's postulates for a causative organism for duodenal ulcer.[69]

Summary

Several lines of evidence suggest there is a consistent, independent association between the presence of chronic vascular *C. pneumoniae* infection and that of atherosclerotic disease, in particular CHD. Anti-*C. pneumoniae* antibody titres tend to be higher in patients with CHD than in controls free of such disease, and a raised titre appears to be a risk factor for developing future cardiovascular events. Furthermore, direct examination of coronary arteries frequently reveals evidence of *C. pneumoniae* organisms or antigens within atheromatous plaques, but rarely within normal tissue close to such lesions or in normal coronary arteries. The organism is more likely to be found in vascular tissue from people who die from CHD than in that from those who die of other (non-cardiac) causes. Limited evidence also suggests that infection may precede or accompany (rather than follow) the early development of atherosclerostic lesions. Despite major methodological difficulties, *C. pneumoniae* has been isolated and cultured from atherosclerotic lesions and deliberate infection can induce the development of such lesions in certain animal models.

These data provide substantial circumstantial evidence that *C. pneumoniae* may contribute to atherogenesis. The next chapter considers mechanisms by which the organism might exert such an effect.

References

1. May J. La intradermoreaccion de Frei en las arteropatias. *Rev Argent Dermatosifil* 1943; **27**: 581–2.
2. Odeh M, Oliven A. Chlamydial infections of the heart. *Eur J Clin Microbiol Infect Dis* 1992; **11**: 885–93.
3. Saikku P, Mattila KJ, Nieminen MS *et al.* Serological evidence of an association of a novel chlamydia, TWAR, with chronic coronary heart disease and acute myocardial infarction. *Lancet* 1988; **ii**: 983–6.
4. Thom DH, Wang SP, Grayston JT *et al. Chlamydia pneumoniae* strain TWAR antibody and angiographically demonstrated coronary artery disease. *Arterioscl Thromb* 1991; **11**: 547–51.
5. Thom DH, Grayston JT, Siscovick DS *et al.* Association of prior infection with *Chlamydia pneumoniae* and angiographically demonstrated coronary artery disease. *JAMA* 1992; **268**: 68–72.
6. Mendall MA, Carrington D, Strachan DP *et al. Chlamydia pneumoniae*: risk factors for seropositivity and association with coronary heart disease. *J Infect* 1995; **30**: 121–8.
7. Patel P, Mendall MA, Carrington D *et al.* Association of *Helicobacter pylori* and *Chlamydia pneumoniae* infections with coronary heart disease and cardiovascular risk factors *BMJ* 1995; **311**: 711–4.
8. Cook PJ, Lip GY, Zarifis J *et al.* Is *Chlamydia pneumoniae* infection associated with acute cardiac ischemic syndromes? *J Am Coll Cardiol* 1996; **807–2**: 324A [abstract].
9. Aceti A, Mazzacurati G, Amendolea M *et al.* Relation of C reactive protein to cardiovascular risk factors: *Helicobacter pylori* and *Chlamydia pneumoniae* infections may account for most acute coronary syndromes. *BMJ* 1996; **313**: 428–9 [letter].
10. Mazzoli S, Tofani N, Fantini A *et al. Chlamydia pneumoniae* antibody response in patients with acute myocardial infarction and their follow-up. *Am Heart J* 1998; **135**: 15–20.
11. Leinonen M, Linnanmaki E, Mattila K *et al.* Circulating immune complexes containing chlamydial lipopolysaccharide in acute myocardial infarction. *Microb Pathog* 1990; **9**: 67–73.
12. Leinonen M. Pathogenetic mechanisms and epidemiology of *Chlamydia pneumoniae. Eur Heart J* 1993; **14** (Suppl. K): 57–61.
13. Saikku P, Leinonen M, Tenkanen L *et al.* Chronic *Chlamydia pneumoniae* infection as a risk factor for coronary heart disease in the Helsinki Heart Study. *Ann Intern Med* 1992; **116**: 273–7.
14. Meittinen H, Lehto S, Saikku P *et al.* Association of *Chlamydia pneumoniae* and acute coronary heart disease events in non-insulin-dependent diabetic and nondiabetic subjects in Finland. *Eur Heart J* 1996; **17**: 682–8.
15. Ossewaarde JM, Feskens EM, DeVries A *et al. Chlamydia pneumoniae* is a risk factor for coronary heart in symptom-free elderly men, but *Helicobacter pylori* and cytomegalovirus are not. *Epidemiol Infect* 1998; **120**: 93–9.
16. Melnick SL, Shahar E, Folsom AR *et al.* Past infection by *Chlamydia pneumoniae* strain TWAR and asymptomatic carotid atherosclerosis. *Am J Med* 1993; **95**: 499–504.
17. Wimmer ML, Sandmann-Strupp R, Saikku P, Harberl RL. Association of chlamydial infection with cerebrovascular disease. *Stroke* 1996; **27**: 2207–10.
18. Cook PJ, Honeybourne D, Lip GH *et al. Chlamydia pneumoniae* antibody titres are significantly associated with acute stroke and transient cerebral ischaemia – The West Birmingham Stroke Project. *Stroke* 1998; **29**: 404–10.
19. Hahn DL, Golubjatnikov R. Smoking is a potential confounder of the *Chlamydia pneumoniae*–coronary disease association. *Arterioscler Thromb* 1992; **12**: 945–7.
20. Karvonen M, Tuomilehto J, Pitkäniemi J, Naukkarinen A, Saikku P. Importance of smoking for *Chlamydia pneumoniae* seropositivity. *Int J Epidemiol* 1994; **23**: 1315–21.

21. Kark JD, Leinonen M, Paltiel O, Saikku P. *Chlamydia pneumoniae* and acute myocardial infarction in Jerusalem. *Int J Epidemiol* 1997; **26**: 730–8.
22. Weiss SM, Roblin PM, Gaydos CA *et al.* Failure to detect *Chlamydia pneumoniae* in coronary atheromas of patients undergoing atherectomy. *J Infect Dis* 1996; **173**: 957–62.
23. Altman R, Rouvier J, Scazziota A *et al.* No association between prior infection with *Chlamydia pneumoniae* and coronary artery disease. *Eur Heart J* 1998; 1643A [abstract].
24. Danesh J, Collins R, Peto R. Chronic infections and coronary heart disease: is there a link? *Lancet* 1997; **350**: 430–6.
25. Gupta S, Camm AJ. *Chlamydia pneumoniae* and coronary heart disease: coincidence, association or causation? *BMJ* 1997; **314**: 1778–9.
26. Shor A, Kuo CC, Patton DL. Detection of *Chlamydia pneumoniae* in coronary arterial fatty streaks and atheromatous plaques. *S Afr Med J* 1992; **82**: 158–61.
27. Kuo CC, Shor A, Campbell LA *et al.* Demonstration of *Chlamydia pneumoniae* in atherosclerotic lesions of coronary arteries. *J Infect Dis* 1993; **167**: 841–9.
28. Davidson M, Kuo CC, Middaugh JP *et al.* Confirmed previous infection with *Chlamydia pneumoniae* (TWAR) and its presence in early coronary atherosclerosis. *Circulation* 1998; **98**: 628–33.
29. Muhlestein JB. Hammond EH, Carlquist JF *et al.* Increased incidence of *Chlamydia* species within coronary arteries of patients with symptomatic atherosclerotic versus other forms of cardiovascular disease. *J Am Coll Cardiol* 1996; **27**: 1555–61.
30. Campbell LA, O'Brien ER, Cappuccio AL *et al.* Detection of *Chlamydia pneumoniae* (TWAR) in human atherectomy tissues. *J Infect Dis* 1995; **172**: 585–8.
31. Ong G, Thomas BJ, Mansfield AO, Davidson BR, Taylor-Robinson D. Detection and widespread distribution of *Chlamydia pneumoniae* in the vascular system and its possible implications. *J Clin Pathol* 1996; **49**: 102–6.
32. Grayston JT, Kuo CC, Coulson AS *et al. Chlamydia pneumoniae* (TWAR) in atherosclerosis of the carotid artery. *Circulation* 1995; **92**: 3397–400.
33. Chiu B, Viira E, Tucker W, Fong IW. *Chlamydia pneumoniae*, cytomegalovirus, and herpes simplex virus in atherosclerosis of the carotid artery. *Circulation* 1997; **96**: 2144–8.
34. Blasi F, Denti F, Erba M *et al.* Detection of *Chlamydia pneumoniae* but not *Helicobacter pylori* in atherosclerotic plaques of aortic aneurysms. *J Clin Microbiol* 1996; **34**: 2766–9.
35. Juvenon JJ, Juvenon T, Laurila A *et al.* Demonstration of *Chlamydia pneumoniae* in the walls of abdominal aortic aneurysms. *J Vasc Surg* 1997; **25**: 499–505.
36. Wong Y, Thomas M, Gallagher PJ *et al.* The prevalence of *Chlamydia pneumoniae* in atherosclerotic and normal blood vessels of patients undergoing redo and first time coronary artery bypass surgery. *J Am Coll Cardiol* 1998; **31**: 146–7A [abstract].
37. Lindholt JS, Ostergard L, Henneberg EW, Fasting H, Anderson P. Failure to demonstrate *Chlamydia pneumoniae* in symptomatic abdominal aortic aneurysms by a nested polymerase chain reaction. *Eur J Vasc Endovasc Surg* 1998; **15**: 161–4.
38. Paterson DL, Hall J, Rasmussen SJ, Timms P. Failure to detect *Chlamydia pneumoniae* in atherosclerotic plaques of Australian patients. *Pathology* 1998; **30**: 169–72.
39. Kuo CC, Grayston JT, Campbell LA *et al. Chlamydia pneumoniae* (TWAR) in coronary arteries of young adults (15–34 years old). *Proc Natl Acad Sci USA* 1995; **92**: 6911–4.
40. Juvenon J, Laurila A, Juvenon T *et al.* Detection of *Chlamydia pneumoniae* in human nonrheumatic stenotic aortic valves. *J Am Coll Cardiol* 1997; **150**: 1054–9.
41. Yang ZP, Kuo CC, Grayston JT. Systemic dissemination of *Chlamydia pneumoniae* following intranasal inoculation in mice. *J Infect Dis* 1995; **171**: 736–8.
42. Jackson LA, Campbell LA, Schmidt RA *et al.* Specificity of detection of *Chlamydia pneumoniae* in cardiovascular atheroma: evaluation of the innocent bystander hypothesis. *Am J Pathol* 1997; **150**: 1785–90.
43. Ramirez JA. Isolation of *Chlamydia pneumoniae* from the coronary artery of a patient with coronary atherosclerosis. The *Chlamydia pneumoniae*/Atherosclerosis Study Group. *Ann Intern Med* 1996; **125**: 979–82.

44. Jackson LA, Campbell LA, Kuo CC *et al.* Isolation of *Chlamydia pneumoniae* from a carotid endarterectomy specimen. *J Infect Dis* 1997; **176**: 292–5.
45. Maass M, Bartels C, Engel PM, Mamat U, Sievers HH. Endovascular presence of viable *Chlamydia pneumoniae* is a common phenomenon in coronary artery disease. *J Am Coll Cardiol* 1998; **31**: 827–32.
46. Naidu BR, Ngeow YF, Kannan P *et al.* Evidence of *Chlamydia pneumoniae* infection obtained by the polymerase chain reaction in patients with acute myocardial infarction and coronary heart disease. *J Infect* 1997; **35**: 199–200 [letter].
47. Condos R, McClune A, Rom WN, Schluger NW. Peripheral-blood-based PCR assay to identify patients with active pulmonary tuberculosis. *Lancet* 1996; **347**: 1082–5.
48. Boman J, Söderberg S, Forsberg J *et al.* High prevalence of *Chlamydia pneumoniae* DNA in peripheral blood mononuclear cells in patients with cardiovascular disease and in middle-aged blood donors. *J Infect Dis* 1998; **178**: 274–7.
49. Wong YK, Dawkins K, Ward ME. Detection of *Chlamydia pneumoniae* DNA circulating in the blood of patients attending for cardiac angiography: preliminary clinical and serological correlates. In: *Chlamydial Infections* (Stephens RS, Byrne GI, Christiansen G *et al.*, eds). International Chlamydial Symposium, San Francisco, USA, 1998; pp. 227–30.
50. Kuo CC, Jackson LA, Campbell L, Grayston JT. *Chlamydia pneumoniae* (TWAR). *Clin Microbiol Rev* 1995; **8**: 451–61.
51. Girjes AA, Carrick FN, Lavin MF. Remarkable sequence relatedness in the DNA encoding the major outer membrane protein of *Chlamydia psittaci* (koala type I) and *Chlamydia pneumoniae. Gene* 1994; **138**: 139–42.
52. Storey C, Lusher M, Yates P, Richmond S. Evidence for *Chlamydia pneumoniae* of non–human origin. *J Gen Microbiol* 1993; **139**: 2621–6.
53. Bell TA, Kuo CC, Wang SP, Grayston JT. Experimental infection of baboons (*Papio cynocephalus anumbis*) with *Chlamydia pneumoniae* strain TWAR. *J Infect* 1989; **19**: 47–9.
54. Holland SM, Taylor H, Gaydos CA, Kappus EW, Quinn TC. Experimental infection with *Chlamydia pneumoniae* in nonhuman primates. *Infect Immun* 1990; **58**: 593–7.
55. Kishimoto T. Studies on *Chlamydia pneumoniae,* strain TWAR infection. I. Experimental infection of *Chlamydia pneumoniae* in mice and serum antibodies against TWAR by MFA. *J Jap Assoc Infect Dis* 1990; **64**: 124–31.
56. Kaukoranta-Tolvanen SS, Laurila AL, Saikku P, Leinonen M, Laitinen K. Experimental infection of *Chlamydia pneumoniae* in mice. *Microb Pathog* 1993; **15**: 293–302.
57. Yang ZP, Kuo CC, Grayston JT. A mouse model of *Chlamydia pneumoniae* strain TWAR pneumonitis. *Infect Immun* 1993; **61**: 2037–40.
58. Yang ZP, Cummings PK, Patton DL, Kuo CC. Ultrastructural lung pathology of experimental *Chlamydia pneumoniae* pneumonitis in mice. *J Infect Dis* 1994; **170**: 464–7.
59. Malinverni R, Kuo CC, Campbell LA, Grayston JT. Reactivation of *Chlamydia pneumoniae* in mice by cortisone. *J Infect Dis* 1995; **172**: 593–4.
60. Laitinen K, Laurila A, Leinonen M, Saikku P. Reactivation of *Chlamydia pneumoniae* infection in mice by cortisone treatment. *Infect Immun* 1996; **64**: 1488–90.
61. Yang ZP, Kuo CC, Grayston JT. Systemic dissemination of *Chlamydia pneumoniae* following intranasal inoculation of mice. *J Infect Dis* 1995; **171**: 736–8.
62. Moazed TC, Kuo CC, Patton DL, Grayston JT, Campbell LA. Experimental rabbit models of *Chlamydia pneumoniae* infection. *Am J Pathol* 1996; **148**: 667–76.
63. Moazed TC, Kuo CC, Grayston JT, Campbell LA. Murine models of *Chlamydia pneumoniae* infection and atherosclerosis. *J Infect Dis* 1997; **175**: 883–90.
64. Fong IW, Chiu B, Viira E *et al.* Rabbit models for *Chlamydia pneumoniae* infection. *J Clin Microbiol* 1997; **35**: 48–52.
65. Laitinen K, Laurila A, Pyhälä L, Leinonen M, Saikku P. *Chlamydia pneumoniae* infection induces inflammatory changes in the aortas of rabbits. *Infect Immun* 1997; **65**: 4832–5.

66. Muhlestein JB, Anderson JL, Hammond EH *et al.* Infection with *Chlamydia pneumoniae* accelerates the development of atherosclerosis and treatment with azithromycin prevents it in a rabbit model. *Circulation* 1998; **97**: 633–6.
67. Moxon ER. Microbes, molecules and man. The Mitchell Lecture 1992. *J Roy Coll Physicians Lond* 1993; **27**: 169–74.
68. Fredericks DN, Relman DA. Sequence–based identification of microbial pathogens: a reconsideration of Koch's postulates. *Clin Microbiol Rev* 1996; **9**: 18–33.
69. Marshall BJ. *Helicobacter pylori* in peptic ulcer: have Koch's postulates been fulfilled? *Ann Med* 1995; **27**: 565–8.
70. Tuazon CU, Varghese PJ, Gaydos CA *et al.* Demonstration of *Chlamydia pneumoniae* in coronary atheroma specimens from young patients with normal cholesterol from the southern part of India. Proceedings of the 7th International Congress of Infectious Diseases 1996; **109.024:** 272 [abstract].
71. Maass M, Krause E, Engel PM, Kruger S. Endovascular presence of *Chlamydia pneumoniae* in patients with haemodynamically effective carotid artery stenosis. *Angiology* 1997; **48**: 699–706.

Chapter 5: Association of *Chlamydia pneumoniae* with atherosclerosis: Potential pathogenetic mechanisms

Introduction

How *Chlamydia pneumoniae* enters atheromatous plaques and whether or not it can cause or contribute to, atherogenesis are not entirely clear. Also, the mounting clinical data suggesting *C. pneumoniae* may have a direct role in atherosclerosis remain largely indirect and do not indicate a particular process by which the organism might exert its effects. This chapter aims to discuss some plausible pathogenetic mechanisms.

Chlamydia pneumoniae transfer within monocyte/macrophage cycle

The presence of *C. pneumoniae* within coronary atheroma suggests that this respiratory pathogen must be conveyed from the lung to cardiac tissue before infection of the cellular components of the coronary arteries can occur.[1] One possibility is that *C. pneumoniae* gains entry to the bloodstream via the macrophage/monocyte system. The organism's ability to multiply in mononuclear cells, particularly alveolar macrophages[2], could ensure transfer from the pulmonary vasculature into the circulation and, thereby, allow systemic dissemination. In support of these ideas, *C. pneumoniae* has been found in various sites in humans including atherosclerotic plaques,[3–5] in the spleen and lymph nodes,[6,7] and in cerebrospinal[8] and synovial fluid.[9] Circumstantial evidence that such dissemination might result in local infection of coronary arteries has been provided by Gaydos *et al.*[10] These workers showed that strains of *C. pneumoniae* could replicate within a cell line of macrophages, human aorta-derived endothelial cells and smooth muscle cells. However, whether or not continuous replication of the organism actually occurs *in vivo* in such cells is not clear.

Persistent pharyngeal carriage of *C. pneumoniae* in patients with CHD

Most infections caused by *C. pneumoniae* are asymptomatic. Gabriel *et al.* have investigated whether patients with coronary heart disease (CHD) have a greater prevalence of *C. pneumoniae* pharyngeal infection (as detected by polymerase chain reaction [PCR]) in the pharynx.[11] They investigated 280 patients with acute and chronic CHD and 102 controls (unmatched for gender and age) without CHD for evidence of *C. pneumoniae* on PCR analysis of pharyngeal specimens and for the presence and of serum anti-*C. pneumoniae* antibodies. Both the prevalence of PCR-positive specimens and anti-*C. pneumoniae* antibodies (IgG ≥1/512) were significantly greater in patients with CHD compared with the controls (36% versus 22%; $p<0.05$; 39% versus 26%; $p<0.05$).

The combined finding of a positive PCR result and elevated serum anti-*C. pneumoniae* antibodies (although not indicative of the presence of viable organisms) strongly suggests ongoing chronic infection. It is postulated that persistent pharyngeal carriage in susceptible subjects could be the source of intermittent dissemination of the organism and help maintain an elevated antibody and general inflammatory response.

Chlamydia pneumoniae-mediated damage in atherogenesis

Foam cell development

A preliminary *in vitro* investigation has shown that *C. pneumoniae* can induce directly the development of foam cells, the lipid-laden macrophages present in the early fatty streak lesion of atherosclerosis.[12] In this study, Kalayoglu *et al.* showed that *C. pneumoniae* infection of human monocyte-derived macrophages, followed by exposure to low-density lipoprotein (LDL)-cholesterol, resulted in marked increase in foam cell formation with accompanying intracellular accumulation of cholesteryl esters. The addition of heparin (which blocks binding of LDL to the LDL receptor) inhibited foam cell development: this suggests that *C. pneumoniae* may be acting by blocking native LDL uptake or metabolism. Interestingly, incubation of macrophages with high levels of *E. coli* LPS induces development of foam cells via similar mechanisms.[13] It is possible that *C. pneumoniae* also modulates macrophage function through its LPS antigen.

The consequences of the uptake of *C. pneumoniae* by macrophages and the mechanisms by which the organism might damage the coronary artery are unclear. The organism may simply reside in the macrophage without causing harmful effects and any association with CHD may be purely coincidental,[1] or due to confounding factors. Alternatively, chronic macrophage infection may contribute directly to local inflammation, development of atheromatous plaques and plaque instability, leading to acute coronary events.[14] For instance, *C. pneumoniae* infection may induce chronic immune activation (mediated by cytokines such as interleukin-1, interleukin-6 and tissue necrosis factor-alpha[15]) that contributes to direct chronic endothelial cell damage or stimulates the synthesis of acute phase proteins, such as fibrinogen[16] and C-reactive protein.[17]

Hypersensitivity and analogies with trachoma

In trachoma, *Chlamydia trachomatis* (an organism closely related to *C. pneumoniae*) causes blindness as a result of fibrosis and scarring that follows conjunctival infiltration by macrophages and lymphocytes.[18] In some people, such fibrosis develops many years after the original infection and may represent a hypersensitivity reaction rather than a direct effect of the organism itself. The effect of *C. pneumoniae* in atherosclerosis may be analogous to trachoma formation, with acute infection and inflammation in the early phases, leading to scarring in later life, in predisposed individuals. Kuo *et al.* found that the chance of identifying *C. pneumoniae* within coronary artery atherosclerotic lesions from autopsy specimens was related inversely to serum anti-*C. pneumoniae* antibody titre, providing indirect evidence that hypersensitivity to *C. pneumoniae* may play a role in atherogenesis.[4] However, these findings were based on a small number of specimens and the antibody titres from haemolysed sera were difficult to evaluate. Furthermore, a more recent study using similar diagnostic techniques, demonstrated *C. pneumoniae* organisms within coronary atherectomy specimens from patients with angina, and found no evidence of an inverse relationship between the likelihood of detecting the organism and the height of the anti-*C. pneumoniae* antibody titre.[19] Similarly, Chiu *et al.* showed no correlation between the presence of *C. pneumoniae* (or cytomegalovirus [CMV]) within carotid atheroma and serum antibody titres.[20] The conflicting findings again emphasise the difficulty in defining the true relationship between a chronic *C. pneumoniae* infection and the anti-*C. pneumoniae* serum antibody level (see Chapter 4).

Potential role of heat shock proteins

Expression of heat shock proteins (HSPs) increases during a variety of conditions (such as heat, nutrient deprivation, infections and inflammatory reactions).[21] Atheromatous vessels contain endogenous human HSP 60[22] and when this protein is expressed by endothelial cells, it can provoke an autoimmune reaction with development of anti-HSP 60 antibodies that lead to endothelial cell damage.[23]

Of interest, a 60 kDa chlamydial HSP has been identified (HSP 60).[24] This protein has close homology with human HSP (which is associated with atherosclerosis[25]). Usually during an infective cycle, chlamydial organisms express basal levels of two major antigens: the major outer membrane protein (MOMP) and the HSP 60. Under certain conditions, the organisms can achieve a state of intracellular, chronic infection in which they remain viable but metabolically quiescent and do not replicate.[26] In such circumstances, HSP 60 production increases substantially, whereas MOMP becomes undetectable.

Kol *et al.*[27] have demonstrated that chlamydia HSP 60 co-localises with its homologue, human HSP 60 within atherosclerotic plaque macrophages. Furthermore, *in vitro*, both human HSP 60 and chlamydial HSP 60 each stimulate enhanced production of TNF-α (a pro-inflammatory cytokine) and matrix metalloproteinase-9 (an enzyme that could degrade connective tissue) by mouse macrophages. On the basis of these results, it has been proposed that macrophages harbouring *C. pneumoniae* infection may trigger these processes and thus promote atherogenesis and precipitate acute coronary events.

Procoagulant effects

Since anti-*C. pneumoniae* antibody titres show a weak correlation with concentrations of important procoagulants such as plasma fibrinogen and factor VIIa,[28] it is possible that chronic infection with this microorganism produces a hypercoaguable state with increased risk of coronary thrombosis. This state could be caused by the monocyte-derived procoagulant, tissue factor.[29]

Possible interaction of *C. pneumoniae* and classical CHD risk factors

The relationship between *C. pneumoniae* infection and established cardiac risk factors could have a crucial bearing on any direct role the organism has in CHD, or could confound any apparent association between the presence of the organism and CHD. It is intriguing, therefore, that *C. pneumoniae* infection is more common in males[30] and that elevated antibodies to *C. pneumoniae* have been associated with hypertension,[31] an atherogenic lipid profile[32] and smoking.[33] It is possible that only a subgroup of the population with certain HLA haplotypes are susceptible to *C. pneumoniae* infection and subsequent development of atherosclerotic disease: this could account for the absence of such disease in only certain individuals exposed to the putative pro-atherogenic pathogen.[34] In support of this notion, a combination of male sex, HLA DR II genotype 13a or 17, elevated levels of lipoprotein (a) and raised anti-IgG *C. pneumoniae* antibody titres (>1/256) have been associated strongly with CHD.[35] Finally, a correlation has also been found between *C. pneumoniae* and elevated levels of fibrinogen[36] and C-reactive protein (CRP), in patients with CHD.[17]

Chlamydia pneumoniae and hypertension

In a case–control study, serum antibodies against *C. pneumoniae* were measured in 131 patients with chronic hypertension and a similar number of controls (matched for age, gender, ethnicity and smoking status) without evidence of cardio-pulmonary disease.[31] Anti-*C. pneumoniae* antibody titres suggestive of chronic infection (defined as IgG 1/64–1/256 or IgA ≥1/8, but IgM ≤1/8 and no rise in IgG) were more prevalent among hypertensive patients, compared with controls (33% versus 17%, p=0.002). On the basis of these findings, the investigators proposed that a chronic *C. pneumoniae* infection might interact with hypertension in promoting development or progression of atherosclerotic vascular disease in hypertensive patients. Such findings have yet to be reproduced in a larger cohort of patients.

Chlamydia pneumoniae and blood lipids

Acute microbial infections can alter lipid metabolism in both experimental animals and humans[37,38] and it is possible that *C. pneumoniae* contributes to atherosclerosis by interacting with serum lipids. Indirect evidence to suggest this comes from cross-sectional study showing a significant association between the presence of IgG anti-*C. pneumoniae* antibodies, elevated triglycerides and reduced high-density-lipoprotein (HDL)-cholesterol levels in a male population in Northern Finland.[39] An extension of this investigation showed that males with a chronic elevation in anti-*C. pneumoniae* antibody titres in serum samples taken 3 years apart (a possible marker of chronic infection) had significantly higher levels of serum total cholesterol and triglycerides, and lower HDL-cholesterol levels compared with males without anti-*C. pneumoniae* antibodies.[32] A potential limitation of the study was that incomplete adjustments were made for potentially confounding determinants of a raised serum cholesterol level.

The LPS of Gram-negative bacteria may alter lipid metabolism,[40] perhaps via induction of cytokines such as IL-1 and TNF-α.[41] Although chlamydial LPS may be of lower virulence than that of enterobacterial organisms,[42] it can induce such cytokine production in blood mononuclear cells *in vitro*.[15] Furthermore, macrophages in atherosclerotic lesions frequently show positive staining with a monoclonal antibody directed against chlamydial LPS.[19,43] It may well be that continuous low-level production of TNF/IL-1 accompanies the persistence of *C. pneumoniae* particles within these cells. This cytokine generation might, in turn, be contributing to an altered, more atherogenic lipid profile.

Chlamydia pneumoniae and fibrinogen

An increased fibrinogen level is both a risk factor for the development of CHD[44] and, like C-reactive protein, a predictor of adverse outcome in unstable angina.[45] Interestingly, one study found an association between raised fibrinogen levels and elevated anti-*C. pneumoniae* IgG antibody titres in men without a history of CHD.[16] Subsequently, a similar association was found between fibrinogen levels and elevated IgA anti-*C. pneumoniae* antibody titres, in individuals with established CHD.[36] Such correlations suggest that a pathogenetic link between chronic *C. pneumoniae* infection and acute and chronic CHD might involve increased activity of thrombotic and inflammatory processes.

Chlamydia pneumoniae and 'the metabolic syndrome'

Chlamydia pneumoniae may promote the effect of the 'metabolic syndrome' (comprising raised body mass index, diabetes mellitus, hypertension and a low HDL-cholesterol level). In one study, patients with serological markers suggesting a chronic *C. pneumoniae* infection plus two or more of determinants of this syndrome were at higher risk of having CHD than were those without such a combination of factors (M Leinonen *et al.*, personal communication). These preliminary findings need further confirmation.

Figure 9: *Chlamydia pneumoniae* in atherothrombosis: Possible mechanisms of damage

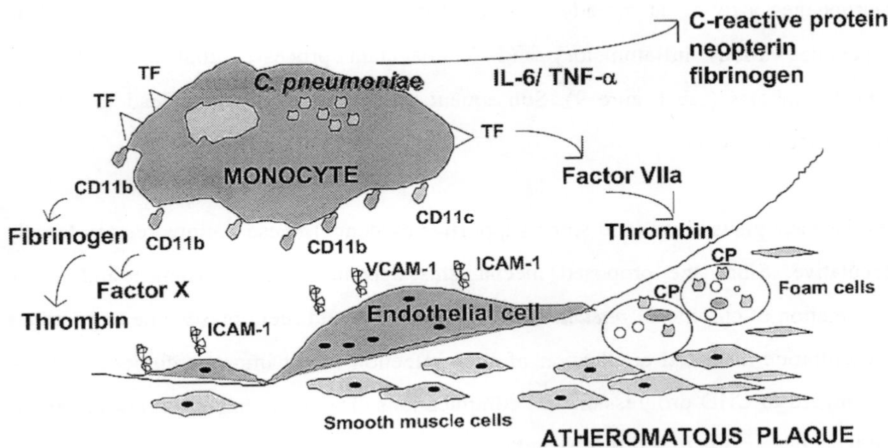

A respiratory infection leading to *C. pneumoniae* (CP) being taken up into the systemic monocyte, to be transported to the coronary circulation. Monocyte activation leading to secretion of cytokines and acute phase proteins, expression of adhesion molecules and up-regulation of tissue factor (TF). The processes either acting independently or interacting to enhance the inflammatory response and perpetuate atherothrombosis. (Reproduced from Gupta S, Camm AJ. Is there an infective aetiology to atherosclerosis? *Drugs Aging* 1998; **13**: 1–7, with permission).

Summary

There are several suggested mechanisms to explain the association between *C. pneumoniae* and atherosclerosis. Monocytes and macrophages may carry the organism from the respiratory tract to the coronary arteries. Subsequent direct endothelial damage caused by a chronic infection of the endothelium (which may be dysfunctional as a result of exposure to toxins derived from cigarette smoking, or to raised serum cholesterol levels) in a genetically predisposed individual may lead to the formation and progression of atherosclerotic lesions. Alternatively, *C. pneumoniae*-infected macrophages arriving at already formed plaque lesions may become 'activated' to perpetuate various inflammatory and procoagulant processes that are central in atherothrombosis (see Figure 9). Subsequent plaque instability may lead to adverse cardiovascular events.

Despite their plausibility (and some supportive evidence), these notions remain largely speculative. Since the proposed mechanisms depend on the existence and active participation of chronic *C. pneumoniae* infection, it would seem reasonable to postulate that antibiotic-mediated eradication of such infection might improve clinical outcome with regard to CHD progression and complications. The next chapter reviews attempts that have been made to test this hypothesis.

References

1. Gupta S, Leatham EW. The relation between *Chlamydia pneumoniae* and atherosclerosis. *Heart* 1997; **77**: 7–8.
2. Black CM, Perez R. *Chlamydia pneumoniae* multiplies within human pulmonary macrophages. *90th Annual Meeting of the American Society for Microbiology*, Washington DC, American Society for Microbiology, 1990, No. D-1, p. 80 [abstract].
3. Kuo CC, Shor A, Campbell LA *et al.* Demonstration of *Chlamydia pneumoniae* in atherosclerotic lesions of coronary arteries. *J Infect Dis* 1993; **167**: 841–9.
4. Grayston JT, Kuo CC, Coulson AS *et al. Chlamydia pneumoniae* (TWAR) in atherosclerosis of the carotid artery. *Circulation* 1995; **92**: 3397–400.
5. Muhlestein JB, Hammond EH, Carlquist JF *et al.* Increased incidence of *Chlamydia* species within the coronary arteries of patients with symptomatic atherosclerotic versus other forms of cardiovascular disease. *J Am Coll Cardiol* 1996; **27**: 1555–61.
6. Yang ZP, Kuo CC, Grayston JT. A mouse model of *Chlamydia pneumoniae* strain pneumonitis. *Infect Immun* 1993; **61**: 2037–40.
7. Yang ZP, Kuo CC, Grayston JT. Systemic dissemination of *Chlamydia pneumoniae* following intranasal inoculation in mice. *J Infect Dis* 1995; **171**: 736–8.
8. Haidl S, Ivarsson S, Bjerre I, Persson K. Guillain–Barré syndrome after *Chlamydia pneumoniae* infection. *N Engl J Med* 1992; **326**: 576–7 [letter].
9. Braun J, Laitko S, Treharne J *et al. Chlamydia pneumoniae* – a new causative agent of reactive arthritis and undifferentiated oligoarthritis. *Ann Rheum Dis* 1994; **53**: 100–5.
10. Gaydos CA, Summersgill JT, Sahney NN, Ramirez JA, Quinn TC. Replication of *Chlamydia pneumoniae in vitro* in human macrophages, endothelial cells, and aortic artery smooth muscle cells. *Infect Immun* 1996; **64**: 1614–20.
11. Gabriel AS, Gnarpe H, Gnarpe J *et al.* The prevalence of chronic *Chlamydia pneumoniae* infection as detected by polymerase chain reaction in pharyngeal samples from patients with ischaemic heart disease. *Eur Heart J* 1998; **19**: 1321–7.
12. Kalayoglu MV, Byrne GI. Induction of macrophage foam cell formation by *Chlamydia pneumoniae*. *J Infect Dis* 1998; **177**: 725–9.
13. Lopes-Virella MF, Klein RL, Stevenson HC. Low density lipoprotein metabolism in human macrophages stimulated with microbial or microbial-related products. *Arteriosclerosis* 1987; **7**: 176–84.
14. Bozovich GE, Gurfinkel EP. *Chlamydia pneumoniae*: More than a bystander in acute coronary syndromes. *Br J Cardiol* 1998; **5**: 84–91.
15. Kaukoranta-Tolvanen SS, Teppo AM, Laitinen K *et al.* Growth of *Chlamydia pneumoniae* in cultured human peripheral blood mononuclear cells and induction of a cytokine response. *Microb Pathog* 1996; **21**: 215–21.
16. Patel P, Carrington D, Strachan DP *et al.* Fibrinogen: a link between chronic infection and coronary heart disease. *Lancet* 1994; **343**: 1634–5.
17. Mendall MA, Patel P, Ballam L, Strachan DP, Northfield TC. C reactive protein and its relation to cardiovascular risk factors: a population based cross sectional study. *BMJ* 1996; **312:** 1061–5.
18. Holland MJ, Bailey RL, Ward ME *et al.* Cell mediated immune responses to *Chlamydia trachomatis* in scarring trachoma. *Proceedings of the European Society of Chlamydial Research* 1992; **2**: 134 [abstract].
19. Campbell LA, O'Brien E, Cappuccio A *et al.* Detection of *Chlamydia pneumoniae* TWAR in human coronary atherectomy tissues. *J Infect Dis* 1995; **172**: 585–8.
20. Chiu B, Viira E, Tucker W, Fong IW. *Chlamydia pneumoniae*, cytomegalovirus and herpes simplex virus in atherosclerosis of the carotid artery. *Circulation* 1997; **96**: 2144–8.
21. Young RA and Elliot TJ. Stress proteins, infection and immune surveillance. *Cell* 1989; **59**: 5–8.

22. Kleindienst R, Xu Q, Willeit J *et al.* Immunology of atherosclerosis: Demonstration of heat shock protein 60 expression and T lymphocytes bearing alpha/beta or gamma/delta receptor in human atherosclerotic lesions. *Am J Pathol* 1993; **142**: 1927–37.
23. Schett G, Xu Q, Amberger A *et al.* Autoantibodies against heat shock protein 60 mediate endothelial cytotoxicity. *J Clin Invest* 1995; **96**: 2569–77.
24. Morrison RP. Chlamydial hsp60 and the immunopathogenesis of chlamydial disease. *Sem Immunol* 1989; **3**: 25–33.
25. Xu Q, Willit J, Marosi M *et al.* Association of serum antibodies to heat shock protein 65 with carotid atherosclerosis. *Lancet* 1993; **341**: 255–9.
26. Beatty WL, Byrne GI, Morrison RP. Repeated and persistent infection with *Chlamydia* and the development of chronic inflammation and disease. *Trends Microbiol* 1994; **2**: 94–8.
27. Kol A, Sukhova GK, Lichtman AH, Libby P. Chlamydial heat shock protein 60 localizes in human atheroma and regulates macrophage tumor necrosis factor-α and matrix metalloproteinase expression. *Circulation* 1998; **98**: 300–7.
28. Patel P, Mendall MA, Carrington D *et al.* Association of *Helicobacter pylori* and *Chlamydia pneumoniae* infections with coronary heart disease and cardiovascular risk factors. *BMJ* 1995; **311**: 711–4.
29. Leatham EW, Bath PM, Tooze JA, Camm AJ. Increased monocyte tissue factor expression in coronary disease. *Br Heart J* 1995; **73**: 10–3.
30. Grayston JT, Wang SP, Campbell LA, Kuo C-C. Current knowledge on *Chlamydia pneumoniae* strain TWAR, an important cause of pneumonia and other acute respiratory diseases. *Eur J Clin Microbiol Infect Dis* 1989; **8**: 191–202.
31. Cook PJ, Lip GY, Davies P *et al. Chlamydia pneumoniae* antibodies in severe essential hypertension. *Hypertension* 1998; **31**: 589–94.
32. Laurila A, Bloigu A, Näyhä S *et al.* Chronic *Chlamydia pneumoniae* infection is associated with a serum lipid profile known to be a risk factor for atherosclerosis. *Arterioscler Thromb Vasc Biol* 1997; **17**: 2910–3.
33. Hahn DL, Golubjatnikov R. Smoking is a potential confounder of the *Chlamydia pneumoniae*-coronary artery disease association. *Arterioscler Thromb* 1992; **12**: 255–60.
34. Libby P, Egan D, Skarlatos S. Roles of infectious agents in atherosclerosis and restenosis: An assessment of the evidence and need for future research. *Circulation* 1997; **96**: 4095–103.
35. Dahlén GH, Boman J, Birgander LS, Lindholm B. Lipoprotein(a), IgG, IgA and IgM antibodies to *Chlamydia pneumoniae* and HLA class II genotype in early coronary artery disease. *Atherosclerosis* 1995; **114**: 165–74.
36. Toss H, Gnarpe J, Gnarpe A *et al.* Increased fibrinogen levels are associated with persistent *Chlamydia pneumoniae* infection in unstable coronary artery disease. *Eur Heart J* 1998; **19**: 570–7.
37. Gallin JI, Kaye D, O'Leary WM. Serum lipids in infection. *N Engl J Med* 1969; **281**: 1081–6.
38. Farshtchi D, Lewis VJ. Effects of three bacterial infections on serum lipids of rabbits. *J Bacteriol* 1968; **95**: 1615–21.
39. Laurila A, Bloigu A, Näyhä S *et al. Chlamydia pneumoniae* antibodies and serum lipids in Finnish males. *BMJ* 1997; **314**: 1456–7.
40. Feingold KR, Pollock AS, Moser AH, Shigenaga JK, Grunfield C. Discordant regulation of proteins of cholesterol metabolism during the acute phase response. *J Lipid Res* 1995; **36**: 1474–82.
41. Feingold KR, Grunfeld C. Tumor necrosis factor-α stimulates hepatic lipogenesis in the rat *in vivo*. *J Clin Invest* 1987; **80**: 184–90.
42. Ingalls RR, Rice PA, Qureshi N *et al.* The inflammatory cytokine response to *Chlamydia trachomatis* infection is endotoxin mediated. *Infect Immun* 1995; **63**: 3125–30.
43. Juveonen J, Juvonen T, Laurila A *et al.* Demonstration of *Chlamydia pneumoniae* in the walls of abdominal aortic aneurysms. *J Vasc Surg* 1997; **25**: 499–505.

44. Meade T, Chakrabati R, Haines A *et al.* Haemostatic function and cardiovascular death: Early results of a prospective study. *Lancet* 1980; **17:** 1050–3.
45. Becker R, Cannon C, Bovill E *et al.* Prognostic value of plasma fibrinogen concentration in patients with unstable angina and non-Q-wave myocardial infarction (TIMI IIIB trial). *Am J Cardiol* 1996; **78:** 142–7.

Chapter 6: Clinical antibiotic trials in coronary heart disease

Introduction

As described in earlier chapters, mounting evidence suggests that *Chlamydia pneumoniae* may have a role in the development and/or progression of atherosclerosis and coronary heart disease (CHD). The data suggesting that *C. pneumoniae* are a potential causative agent in this setting far exceeds that for other proposed infectious agents, and is based on the findings of seroepidemiological studies, direct examination of atheromatous plaque specimens, *in vitro* experiments and animal models. A further important line of evidence has been the results of preliminary anti-chlamydial antibiotic intervention studies in CHD.[1,2] This chapter focuses on the potential role of such antimicrobial therapy in the secondary prevention of CHD. The findings of preliminary pilot studies are reviewed, as are the aims and controversies surrounding subsequent large-scale, prospective intervention trials now in progress.

The choice of macrolide therapy in intervention trials

The first two pilot intervention trials in CHD used macrolide antibiotics, namely azithromycin[1] and roxithromycin.[2] Furthermore, the ongoing large-scale prospective trials are using azithromycin in the treatment arm of the studies. The reasons for choosing azithromycin as the trial antibiotic in this setting merit discussion.

Azithromycin is the first azalide, a new class of macrolide antibiotics. It has a distinctive pharmacokinetic profile. For example, after dosing, there is extensive absorption and distribution of the drug, such that tissue concentrations may be 10–100 times serum levels (see Figure 10).[3] Also, although plasma clearance of the drug is rapid, release from tissues is slow and the drug's serum half-life is long (68 hours).

Furthermore, the unchanged drug can be detected in the urine for up to 14 days after a single dose. Azithromycin is actively and avidly taken up by macrophages and polymorphonuclear neutrophils and transported to sites of infection. Again, its release from tissues is very slow. Evidence for this comes from a study in which patients undergoing bronchoscopy took a single oral 500mg dose of azithromycin; the drug was subsequently detectable in sputum, bronchial mucosa, epithelial lining fluid and alveolar macrophages up to 96 hours later.[4] (See Figure 11.)

Azithromycin's extensive tissue penetration and high intracellular concentrations suggest that it might be useful treatment in infections caused by sensitive intracellular pathogens, such as Chlamydiae. Azithromycin has been shown to be highly effective against *C. pneumoniae*, in both *in vitro* and clinical studies,[5] and has an excellent tolerability record. The convenient short-course regimen of 500mg once daily for 3 days facilitates adherence to therapy. In addition, the experience of safe, long-term usage of azithromycin is vast, especially in the prophylactic treatment of disseminated *Mycobacterium avium* complex disease in HIV-infected patients, who are often given therapy for as long as 2 years.[6]

In summary, the favourable therapeutic properties of azithromycin include its availability in a short-course regimen, the sustained intra-macrophage concentrations associated with its use, the drug's potency against *C. pneumoniae* and its excellent tolerability. These characteristics make it a particularly suitable choice of antibiotic in intervention trials in patients with CHD.

Figure 10: High azithromycin concentration within macrophages

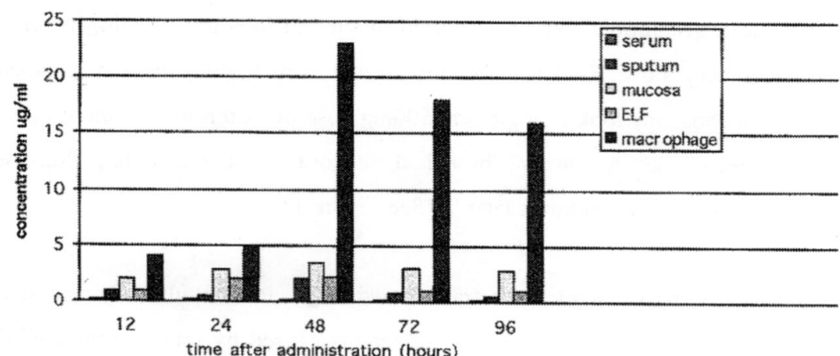

Mean azithromycin concentration following administration of a single 500mg oral dose to patients undergoing bronchoscopy. ELF = epithelial lining fluid. (Adapted from Baldwin DR, Wise R, Andrew JM *et al.* Azithromycin concentrations at the sites of pulmonary infection. *Eur Resp J* 1990; **3:** 886–90, with permission.)

Figure 11: High azithromycin penetration and concentration within tissues

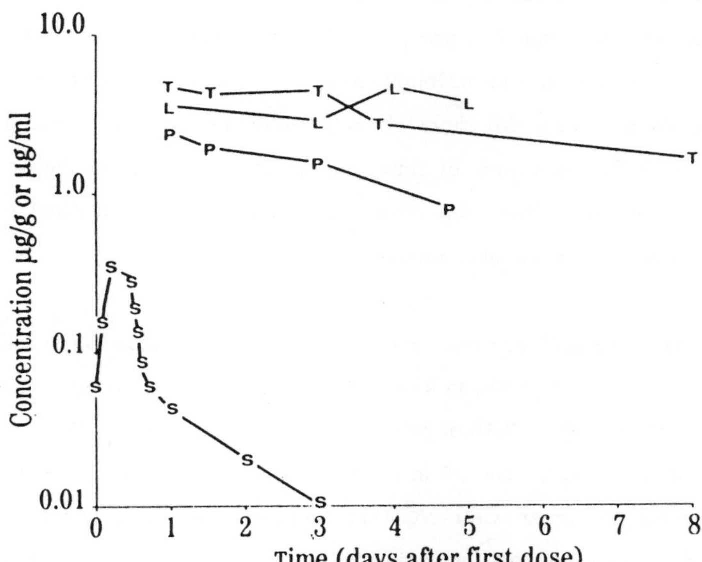

Mean tissue concentration of azithromycin after administration of a single 500mg dose. L = lung; P = prostate; S = serum; T = tonsil. (Adapted from Foulds G, Shepard RM, Johnson RB *et al.* The pharmacokinetics of azithromycin in human serum and tissue. *J Antimicrob Chemother* 1990; **25** (Suppl A): 73–82, with permission.)

Pilot antibiotic studies

St George's study: azithromycin in male survivors of MI

In a randomised, placebo-controlled study, azithromycin (500mg once daily for 3 or 6 days) was given to a series of male survivors of myocardinal infarction (MI) with stable elevated anti-*C. pneumoniae* antibody titres (i.e. two raised IgG titres of ≥1/64, taken 3 months apart).[7] The primary hypothesis under test was that *C. pneumoniae* infection may have a pathogenetic role in atherogenesis via enhanced activation of serum and monocyte markers. A reduction in the levels of such activation markers following treatment with an anti-chlamydial antibiotic could provide indirect evidence that *C. pneumoniae* does indeed act through such a mechanism. The study also assessed whether an elevated anti-*C. pneumoniae* antibody titre predicted further adverse cardiovascular events (at a mean follow-up of 18 months), in a consecutive series of 220 males who had had an MI (from whom the antibiotic intervention trial participants were drawn).[1] The incidence of future cardiovascular events in the subgroup of patients with elevated titres who were randomised (in a double-blind fashion) to azithromycin or placebo was also observed.

By 6 months in the antibiotic intervention trial, the anti-*C. pneumoniae* antibody titre had fallen from ≥1/64 to <1/16 in 43% (17/40) of patients who received azithromycin compared with only 10% (2/20) of patients taking placebo (p=0.02). Subjects receiving azithromycin had a significant fall in levels of certain serum and monocyte activation markers (monocyte integrins CD11b/CD11c, fibrinogen and leucocyte count; p<0.05).[7] These findings help support the hypothesis that *C. pneumoniae* contributes to the progression of atherosclerosis via up-regulation of inflammatory markers.

The study also showed that the higher the baseline anti-*C. pneumoniae* antibody titre, the greater the risk of experiencing an adverse cardiovascular event, an association which persisted following correction for potential confounding variables. (See Tables 8 and 9.)

There was a fourfold higher risk of experiencing adverse cardiovascular events among the group with elevated *C. pneumoniae* titres compared with the group with negative serology (odds ratio 4.2 [95% CI 1.2–15.5; p=0.03]). For the high-titre group receiving antibiotic therapy, the adjusted odds ratio was 0.9 (0.2–4.6; p=ns).

Table 8: Patient characteristics and incidence of cardiovascular events at a mean of 18±4 months of follow-up

Group	Cp–ve (*n*=59)	Cp-I (*n*=74)	Cp+ve-NR (*n*=20)	Cp+ve-P (*n*=20)	Cp+ve-A (*n*=40)
Age, *y* (mean±SD	63±8	61±9	63±9	60±9	58±7
Diabetes mellitus, *n* (%)	6 (10)	9 (12)	6 (30)	8 (40)	12 (30)
Hypertension, *n* (%)	15 (25)	9 (12)	3 (15)	4 (20)	7 (18)
Previous PTCA or CABG, *n* (%)	12 (20)	20 (27)	8 (40)	6 (30)	12 (30)
Hyperlipidemia, *n* (%)	23 (39)	31 (42)	10 (50)	7 (35)	18 (45)
Smoking (past), *n* (%)	39 (66)	40 (54)	14 (70)	10 (50)	21 (53)
Smoking (current), *n* (%)	7 (12)	16 (22)	3 (15)	5 (25)	14 (35)
Months since MI, mean±SD	44±32	44±27	46±32	39±24	47±32
Anterior MI, %	53	53	50	58	53
Ejection fraction, %	41±14	45±13	41±19	47±14	48±14
Adverse cardiovascular events, *n*					
Death	0	0	1	1	1
Unstable angina/MI	0	7	4	4	2
PTCA/CABG	4	4	1	0	0
Total (%)	4 (7)	11 (15)	6 (30)	5 (25)	3 (8)
χ^2 versus Cp–ve	–	2.1	7.3	4.9	0.9
P	–	0.1	0.007	0.03	NS

Cp = *Chlamydia pneumoniae*. Cp–ve = seronegative group of patients; Cp-I = group with intermediate antibody titres; Cp+ve-NR/P = group with elevated antibody titres either randomized to placebo or not randomized; Cp+ve-A = group with elevated antibody titres randomized to azithromycin; CABG = coronary artery bypass surgery; PTCA = percutaneous transluminal coronary angioplasty. (From Gupta S, Leatham EW, Carrington D *et al.* Elevated *Chlamydia pneumoniae* antibodies, cardiovascular events and azithromycin in male survivors of myocardial infarction. *Circulation* 1997; **96**: 404–17, with permission.)

Table 9: Odds ratios for cardiovascular events in seronegative and seropositive patient groups

Group	Total CV Events, *n* (%)	Unadjusted OR (95% CI)	Adjusted OR (95% CI)
Cp–ve (*n*=59)	4 (7)		
Cp-I (*n*=74)	1 (15)	2.4 (0.7–8.0)	2.0 (0.6–6.8)
Cp+ve-NR/P (*n*=40)	11 (28)	5.2 (1.5–17.8)[a]	5.2 (1.5–17.8)[b]
Cp+ve-A (*n*=40)	3 (8)	1.1 (0.2–5.3)	0.9 (0.2–4.6)

See Table 8 for explanation of group designations.
Comparisons of cardiovascular (CV) events are all groups relative to group Cp–ve [expressed as OR (95% confidence interval (CI)]. Adjusted OR calculated after controlling for the following variables: age, diabetes mellitus, smoking status, hypertension, hyperlipidemia and previous coronary revascularization. [a]P=0.008; [b]P=0.03 versus group Cp–ve. (From Gupta S, Leatham EW, Carrington D *et al.* Elevated *Chlamydia pneumoniae* antibodies, cardiovascular events and azithromycin in male survivors of myocardial infarction. *Circulation* 1997; **96**: 404–17, with permission.)

The study findings suggest that anti-*C. pneumoniae* antibody titre may help predict the risk of further cardiovascular events in male survivors of MI, and that azithromycin might reduce this risk. The trial results do not, however, help to distinguish conclusively between an anti-*C. pneumoniae* effect of azithromycin, or an non-antimicrobial effect (such as anti-inflammatory actions). Nevertheless, it is interesting to note that a greater proportion of patients receiving azithromycin had a fall in their anti-*C. pneumoniae* antibody titres at 6 months than those assigned to placebo, perhaps suggesting that the antibiotic may have been suppressing infection, or accelerating clearance of antibodies. The small size of the study dictates that a much larger purpose-designed, prospective trial would be needed to confirm the preliminary findings.

Roxithromycin in Ischaemic Syndromes (ROXIS) study

The aim of the ROXIS study[2] (another pilot, randomised, placebo-controlled intervention trial) was to assess whether the anti-chlamydial antibiotic, roxithromycin (150 mg twice daily, for 30 days) could reduce the incidence of recurrent ischaemic events in 205 patients who had presented with acute coronary syndromes. Conventional anti-anginal therapy (aspirin, heparin and beta-blockers) was continued in all patients. There was a significant reduction in combined ischaemic events (composite endpoint: recurrent ischaemia, MI or ischaemic death) at day 31 in the patients randomised to roxithromycin compared with the placebo group (two versus nine events, $p=0.03$ unadjusted, $p=0.06$ adjusted) (see Table 10). Follow-up results of this study suggest that the benefit derived from therapy may be independent of baseline anti-*C. pneumoniae* IgG antibody serology (E Gurfinkel, personal communication). An anti-inflammatory, 'plaque-stabilising' effect of macrolide therapy is one postulated mechanism to explain the clinical results of this trial. Alternatively, roxithromycin therapy may have suppressed the reactivation of a chronic *C. pneumoniae* infection within the atherosclerotic plaque.

Table 10: Cardiovascular events occurring from 72 hours to day 31 (ROXIS Trial)

	Placebo (*n*=93) (%)	**Roxithromycin (*n*=93) (%)**	***P* Unadjusted[a]**	**Adjusted[b]**
Recurrent angina	5 (5)	1 (1%)	0.211	0.633
Acute mycocardial infarction	2 (2)	0	0.497	0.9
Death	2 (2)	0	0.497	0.9
Double endpoint[c]	4 (4)	0	0.121	0.242
Triple endpoint[d]	9 (10)	1 (1%)	0.018	0.036

[a]Fisher's exact test; [b]Bonferroni-corrected Fisher's exact test; [c]acute myocardial plus ischaemic death; [d]severe recurrent angina, plus acute myocardial infarction, plus ischaemic death. (From Gurfinkel E, Bozovich G, Daroca A, Beck E, Mautner B. Randomised trial of roxithromycin in non-Q-wave coronary syndromes: ROXIS pilot study. *Lancet* 1997; **350**: 404–17, with permission.)

Trial of doxycycline in bypass-surgery patients

In a small, randomised, placebo-controlled study, doxycycline therapy was investigated in 34 non-smoking males who had had previous coronary artery bypass surgery (CABG).[8] After 4 months of trial treatment, no significant differences were noted in anti-*C. pneumoniae* antibody titres, laboratory risk factors for CHD (including lipids, fibrinogen and thrombin fragments) or nitric oxide production (as determined by forearm blood flow responses) between the doxycycline-treated and placebo-treated groups. The investigators acknowledged that the study numbers were too small to assess any clinical effects, that antibiotic monotherapy may not be sufficient to eradicate a chronic chlamydial infection and that antibody serology itself may not be an appropriate marker for confirming the presence of such infection.

Do anti-inflammatory actions of macrolides account for the clinical benefits?

The two preliminary trials of macrolide therapy in CHD have shown a potential clinical benefit in the antibiotic-treated groups,[1,2] with reduction in the incidence of adverse cardiovascular events. These effects may have resulted from an action against *C. pneumoniae* (more likely to be suppression of active infection, rather than its complete eradication, given the short courses of therapy used) or may reflect an independent anti-inflammatory effect of azithromycin or roxithromycin. Several studies have demonstrated that macrolides antibiotics have anti-inflammatory actions. *In vitro*, macrolides inhibit the proliferation of peripheral blood mononuclear cells,[9] reduce the formation of superoxide by neutrophils and inhibit the release of cytokines.[10,11] In addition, investigation by Martin *et al.* showed that *in vitro*, roxithromycin (but not tetracycline) produced a significant reduction in whole-cell conductance of macrophages via blockade of the large-conductance potassium channel.[12] Whether this *in vitro* effect could translate into an *in vivo* benefits (for example, by suppression of macrophage activity and rendering the atherosclerotic plaque less vulnerable to rupture) needs to be tested in a clinical trial.

Ongoing prospective antibiotic studies

The publication of the first two pilot studies of macrolide therapy in the prevention of coronary events generated widespread scientific interest. Large-scale, prospective antibiotic trials in this setting are underway; the aims and designs of major studies are described briefly below.

'Weekly Intervention with Zithromax against Atherosclerotic-Related Disorders' (WIZARD) study

The WIZARD study, a multi-centre prospective trial, was launched in Autumn 1997 (M Dunne, personal communication). It has randomised around 3500 patients who have had an MI more than 6 weeks previously, and who have positive anti-*C. pneumoniae* serology (≥1/16 IgG), to receive either an acute 3-day course of azithromycin (600mg/day) followed by a chronic 3-month course of the antibiotic (600mg, given weekly), or to receive placebo throughout. The primary aim of the study is to assess whether antibiotic therapy can reduce total cardiovascular events over a 2.5-year follow-up period. The overall duration of antibiotic therapy is arbitrary, but based on a logical rationale. An acute course of azithromycin may treat any active *C. pneumoniae* infection, and perhaps stabilise atherosclerotic plaques. An ongoing chronic course of therapy would be needed to attempt eradication of a deep-seated infection – in which the organism might exhibit a cyclical pattern of remaining quiescent for long periods, and emerging intermittently in an unpredictable active phase. In the active phase, an adequate local concentration of the drug would be necessary, hence the use of a weekly regimen. The WIZARD study may not be able to differentiate between any non-antimicrobial action of the antibiotic and antibacterial effects, since this study includes only anti-*C. pneumoniae* seropositive patients. Provision is made to assess changes in anti-*C. pneumoniae* titres and inflammatory markers during the course of the study. Trial cardiovascular endpoints are currently being reviewed.

'Might Azithromycin Reduce Bypass-List Events?' (MARBLE) study

An intrinsic limitation of the British National Health Service system is the reality of waiting lists for coronary revascularisation procedures. In an average tertiary cardiothoracic unit, for instance, around 700–800 patients with severe CHD will be on a typical waiting list for CABG procedures. These people can expect to wait for up to 12 months for surgery. Such patients often have cardiovascular events during the waiting period (including readmission with unstable angina or MI[13]) or other evidence of worsening coronary artery disease.[14] The MARBLE study is a prospective, double-blind antibiotic trial that aims to randomise such 'CABG-waiters' to an azithromycin regimen identical to that of the WIZARD study or to placebo (irrespective of baseline serum anti-*C. pneumoniae* antibody titre), and to assess effects on the total number of cardiovascular events occurring during the period waiting for CABG.[14] At the time of operation, a proportion (20–25%) of these patients are likely to undergo coronary endarterectomy procedures. Samples of coronary arteries taken at this time will be examined for presence of *C. pneumoniae*, and correlations made with serology, inflammatory markers and any effects of antibiotic treatment. The results of the MARBLE study, if positive, may provide data on the relationship between antibiotic treatment and effects of infection within coronary arteries, and, moreover, could have major public health and socioeconomic ramifications for the UK.

'Azithromycin in Coronary Artery Disease: Elimination of Myocardial Infection with *Chlamydia*' (ACADEMIC) study

The ACADEMIC study is a small, double-blind, randomised secondary prevention trial to test whether or not azithromycin reduces serum levels of systemic markers of inflammation, anti-*C. pneumoniae* antibody titres or vascular events in patients with symptomatic CHD (post-MI or angiographically confirmed disease). In all, 150 patients have been randomised to a 3-month course of azithromycin and 150 to placebo. Preliminary results (at 6 months) show a significant stabilisation of C-reactive protein (CRP) and interleukin-6 (IL-6) levels and a trend toward stabilisation of interleukin-1 levels.[16] No difference has been demonstrated in laboratory markers, antibody titres or clinical cardiovascular events at 3 or 6 months, for the latter two endpoints – perhaps not surprisingly given the study's small size. The primary clinical endpoint (total cardiovascular events) evaluation will be at a 2-year follow-up point.

'South Thames Antibiotics in Myocardial Infarction and Angina' (STAMINA) study

In the STAMINA study, 600 patients with acute coronary syndromes are being randomised to either an azithromycin-based regimen, an amoxycillin-based regimen or placebo (with the aim of treating both *H. pylori* and *C. pneumoniae* infections), to assess consequent effects of such therapy on serological markers of infection, inflammatory markers (fibrinogen, CRP, IL-6) and, secondarily, on clinical cardiovascular events (A Stone, personal communication).

'CROatian Azithromycin in Atherosclerosis Study' (CROAATS)

The CROAATS is a placebo-controlled, randomised trial involving 400 survivours of MI (J Culic, personal communication). The primary aim is to investigate the effects of taking azithromycin 500mg daily for 3 days in three cycles (days 1–3, 10–12 and 20-22) on total cardiovacular events over a 18-month follow-up period. Secondary endpoints include effects of therapy on serological markers, inflammatory and procoagulant mediators. Only patients with positive anti-*C. pneumoniae* antibody titres will be randomised to azithromycin or placebo. However, screened, non-randomised (i.e. seronegative) patients will also be observed prospectively for future cardiovascular events.

'Azithromycin and Coronary Events Study' (ACES)

ACES is planned to be a multi-centre, placebo-controlled trial. The study group will comprise 4000 adults with established CHD. Subjects will be randomised to take either azithromycin (600mg) or placebo, once weekly for 1 year, irrespective of their baseline anti-*C. pneumoniae* antibody titre. The composite primary endpoint will be cardiovascular death, non-fatal MI or hospitalisation for unstable angina and revascularisation procedures. The monitoring period will average 4 years (JT Grayston, personal communication).

Potential limitations of the antibiotic studies

In the understandable drive to complete the large antibiotic intervention trials promptly, certain important issues could be inadvertently overlooked. Such points include: difficulties in confirming chronic *C. pneumoniae* infection, precise characterisation of any subgroups of patients likely to benefit from (or to be harmed by) antibiotic therapy, potential effects of reinfection with *C. pneumoniae* and the possible confounding by other infections.[17] The potential implications of widespread use of broad-spectrum antibiotics in the community and the risk of increased antibiotic resistance, a very topical issue, also needs careful consideration and risk–benefit evaluation.

It is also possible that negative findings in the ongoing prospective trials may fail to provide definitive evidence that either *C. pneumoniae* or antimicrobial therapy have no role in CHD. This could be the case if there is an under-powering of the trials, incomplete eradiaction of any *C. pneumoniae* infection or an inadequate follow-up time in the setting of a delayed therapeutic benefit.

Antimicrobial resistance

International agencies (including the World Health Organization) are highlighting and addressing the increasing problem of widespread antimicrobial resistance.[18] There is evidence suggesting that up to 75% of total antibiotic use is of questionable therapeutic value, and it is not unusual to find organisms insensitive to multiple different antibiotics. Strategies, such as increasing surveillance, education and application of evidence-based guidelines on prescribing, are being implemented to limit the development and spread of resistance. Further research is also crucial to improve our understanding of the evolution of resistance, its spread in the community and effective mechanisms for its control. The current focus on the potential use of antibiotics in the management of CHD raises inevitable concerns over the effects on antimicrobial resistance of widespread (and prolonged) usage of broad-spectrum antibiotics in a new clinical arena.

How the antibiotic studies should help

Despite their limitations, the ongoing antibiotic trials are likely to increase our understanding of the role of infection and antimicrobials in CHD. Should the trials confirm the results of the pilot studies, antibiotic treatment of chronic *C. pneumoniae* infection could have major therapeutic implications and potentially help reduce the burden of the epidemic of CHD which persists, despite other advances in risk factor modification and coronary interventions. The provision of a relatively inexpensive form of secondary prevention could be particularly beneficial to countries in Eastern Europe and the developing world that are seeing a disproportionate increase in the incidence of CHD. Such results should also help to determine the overall risk–benefit ratio of chronic antibiotic usage in CHD and thereby limit prescribing practice that could otherwise unnecessarily increase levels of antimicrobial resistance. On the other hand, negative results from the trials would help prevent a well-intentioned but inappropriate and potentially harmful widespread use of broad-spectrum antibiotics.

Summary

Macrolide antibiotics are well-established treatments for *C. pneumoniae* infection. Such drugs are, therefore, a logical choice in studies testing whether therapy targeted at presumed (or possible) chronic *C. pneumoniae* improves clinical outlook in CHD. Pilot antibiotic studies (using azithromycin and roxithromycin) suggest that such intervention may indeed help prevent cardiovascular events in patients with established CHD. Larger randomised, controlled trials should help establish definitively whether antibiotic therapy would be a useful treatment strategy in such patients. They may also help in clarifying the nature of the inter-relationship between chronic vascular *C. pneumoniae* infection and atherosclerotic disease.

References

1. Gupta S, Leatham EW, Carrington D *et al.* Elevated *Chlamydia pneumoniae* antibodies, cardiovascular events and azithromycin in male survivors of myocardial infarction. *Circulation* 1997; **96**: 404–17.
2. Gurfinkel E, Bozovich G, Daroca A, Beck E, Mautner B. Randomised trial of roxithromycin in non-Q-wave coronary syndromes: ROXIS pilot study. *Lancet* 1997; **350**: 404–17.
3. Foulds G, Shepard RM, Johnson RB. The pharmacokinetics of azithromycin in human serum and tissue. *J Antimicrob Chemother* 1990; **25** (Suppl A): 73–82.
4. Baldwin DR, Wise R, Andrews JM, Ashby D, Honeybourne D. Azithromycin concentrations at the sites of pulmonary infection. *Eur Resp J* 1990; **3**: 886–90.
5. Rizzato G, Montemurro L, Fraioli P *et al.* Efficacy of a three-day course of azithromycin in moderately severe community-acquired pneumonia. *Eur Respir J* 1995; **8**: 398–402.
6. Havlir DV, Dubé MP, Sattler FR *et al.* Prophylaxis against disseminated *Mycobacterium avium* complex with weekly azithromycin, daily rifabutin, or both. *N Engl J Med* 1996; **335**: 392–8.
7. Gupta S, Leatham EW, Carrington D *et al.* The effect of azithromycin in post myocardial infarction patients with elevated *Chlamydia pneumoniae* antibody titers. *J Am Coll Cardiol* 1997; **755**: 209 [abstract].
8. Sinisalo J, Mattila K, Nieminen MS *et al.* The effect of prolonged doxycycline therapy on *Chlamydia pneumoniae* serological markers, coronary heart disease risk factors and forearm basal nitric oxide production. *J Antimicrob Chemother* 1998; **41**: 85–92.
9. Roche Y, Gougerot-Pocidalo M-A, Forest N, Pocidalo J-J. Macrolides and immunity: Effects of erythromycin and spiramycin on human mononuclear cell proliferation. *J Antimicrob Chemother* 1986; **17**: 195–203.
10. Anderson R. Erythromycin and roxithromycin potentiate human neutrophil locomotion *in vitro* by inhibition of leukoattractant-activated superoxide generation and auto-oxidation. *J Infect Dis* 1989; **159**: 966–73.
11. Konno S, Adachi M, Asano K, Okomoto K, Takahashi T. Anti-allergic activity of roxithromycin: inhibition of interleukin-5 production from mouse T-lymphocytes. *Life Sci* 1993; **52**: 25–30.
12. Martin D, Bursill J, Qui MR, Breit SN, Campbell T. Alternative hypothesis for efficacy of macrolides in acute coronary syndromes. *Lancet* 1998; **351**: 1858–9.
13. Bengston A, Karlsson T, Hjalmarson Å, Herlitz J. Complications prior to revascularisation among patients waiting for coronary artery bypass grafting and percutaneous transluminal coronary angioplasty. *Eur Heart J* 1996; **17**: 1846–51.
14. Kaski JC, Chester MR, Chen L, Katritsis D. Rapid angiographic progression of coronary artery disease in patients with angina pectoris. *Circulation* 1995; **92**: 2058–65.
15. Gupta S, Camm AJ. *Chlamydia pneumoniae*, antimicrobial therapy and coronary heart disease: a critical overview. *Coron Artery Dis* 1998; **9**: 339–43.
16. Anderson JL, Muhlestein JB. Azithromycin in coronary artery disease: Elimination of myocardial infection with *Chlamydia.* ACADEMIC study. Presented at 47th Scientific session of the American College of Cardiology meeting, Atlanta, Georgia, USA, 1998.
17. Gupta S, Kaski JC, Camm AJ. Antibiotics therapy and coronary heart disease: hype versus hope? *Br J Cardiol* 1998; **5**: 65–6.
18. Wise R, Hart T, Cars D *et al.* Antimicrobial resistance. *BMJ* 1998; **317**: 609–10.

Chapter 7: A perspective on *Chlamydia pneumoniae* and coronary heart disease

There is a consistent association between evidence of the presence of *Chlamydia pneumoniae* infection and coronary heart disease (CHD), but a causal relationship between the organism and atherogenesis has not been established[1] (See Table 11). Since the original report in 1988 suggesting that *C. pneumoniae* was linked with CHD,[2] there has been, understandably, a rather mixed response from the scientific community, including doubt, speculation, excitement and intense research. The original observations have led to numerous follow-up investigations in many countries. These included: seroepidemiological studies showing associations between anti-*C. pneumoniae* antibodies and CHD,[3] positive identification of the organism within,[4] and its culture from, atheroma;[5–7] development of animal models of *C. pneumoniae*-induced atherogenesis;[8–10] *in vitro* studies providing evidence of an 'infectious' basis for atherogenesis; and clinical intervention secondary prevention studies using anti-chlamydial antibiotics.[11,12] The international nature of research in this field can be seen from the map in Figure 12, which highlights countries where important studies have been carried out or are ongoing.

Table 11: Lines of evidence linking *C. pneumoniae* with atherosclerosis

Lines of evidence
Consistent serological link with vascular diseases
Infection of vascular cells *in vitro*
Identification and culture from atheroma
Induction of atherosclerosis in animal models
Potential therapeutic benefit of anti-chlamydial antibiotics

Figure 12: *Chlamydia pneumoniae* and atherosclerosis: A global phenomenon?

Country	Study	Country	Study
Finland	Saikku *et al*, 1988	Japan	Miyashita *et al*, 1998
USA	Thom *et al*, 1992	Australia	Martin *et al*, 1998
South Africa	Shor *et al*, 1992	Austria	Palisek-Kiss *et al*, 1998
UK	Mendall *et al*, 1995	France	Tier et al, 1998
Sweden	Dahlen *et al*, 1995	Hungary	Gonczol et al, 1998
Netherlands	Ossewaarde *et al*, 1995	Denmark	Lindholt et al, 1998
Greece	Gounaris *et al*, 1995	Ireland	(in progress)
India	Tuazon *et al*, 1996	Scotland	(in progress)
Italy	Aceti *et al*, 1996	Croatia	(in progress)
Argentina	Gurfinkel *et al*, 1997	Turkey	(in progress)
Malaysia	Naidu *et al*, 1997	Saudi Arabia	(in progress)
Germany	Maass *et al*, 1997	Cameroon	(in progress)
Mexico	Breceda *et al*, 1997	China	(in progress)
Canada	Fong *et al*, 1997	Switzerland	(in progress)
Hong Kong	Thomas *et al*, 1997	Belgium	(in progress)
Norway	Ånestad *et al*, 1997		

Use of anti-chlamydial antibiotics and fall in cardiovascular disease mortality

It is of additional interest that some investigators have noted that there is a positive epidemiological correlation between the introduction of anti-chlamydial antibiotics and the decline in cardiovascular disease (CVD) mortality seen in certain countries over the last 3–4 decades. For example, Ånestad *et al.* compared mortality rates from CVD in Norway with some lifestyle risk factors (i.e. dietary fat intake and cigarette smoking) and the consumption of tetracycline.[14] They showed that CVD mortality rates peaked in 1961–65 – but both fat intake and smoking rates in the community remained high for at least another decade. On the other hand, increasing usage of tetracycline after the drug was licensed in Norway in 1954 mirrored a temporal fall in CVD mortality (see Figure 13). Saikku et al have made similar observations, relating the declining mortality from CHD in Finland to the introduction of erythromycin and other macrolides (P Saikku, personal communication].

Figure 13: Cardiovascular disease deaths in Norway, dietary fat and consumption of tetracycline

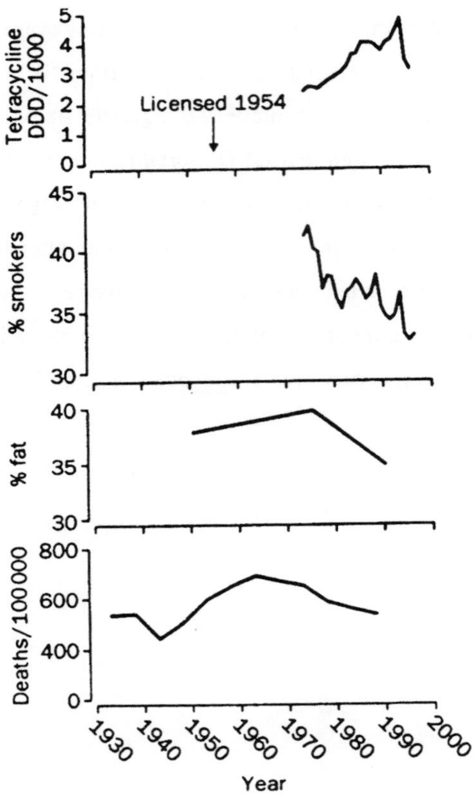

Deaths per 100,000 population from cardiovascular diseases: CVD according to ICD9 (International Classification of Diseases, 9th revision) codes 390–459. Standardised on the basis of age at December 31, 1990, % of total energy from fat (g fat per 10 MJ), % of smokers (16–74 years), and consumption of tetracycline in defined daily doses (DDD) per 1000. (Data obtained from Statistics Norway, Norwegian Nutritional Council, National Council of Tobacco and Health, and Norwegian Medicinal Depot). (Reproduced from Ånestad G, Scheel G, Hugnes O. Chronic infections and coronary heart disease. Lancet 1997; 350: 1028 [letter], with permission.)

Despite all these research findings, our understanding of the organism's natural history and role in chronic disease processes, such as atherosclerosis, is incomplete. The organism is difficult to culture and, therefore, diagnosis of infection has relied largely on indirect methods, such as checking for anti-*C. pneumoniae* antibodies using microimmunofluorescence assays. The precise relationship between anti-*C. pneumoniae* antibody titres and infection status (in patients with or without CHD) and any serological criteria for eradication of *C. pneumoniae* infection remain undefined. Also, published seroepidemiological studies have used arbitrarily selected anti-*C. pneumoniae* antibody titre cut-off points to define seropositivity and there is a lack of reliable and reproducible methods of detecting the organism's antigens.[3] Stringent criteria for the definition and diagnosis of chronic *C. pneumoniae* infection in CHD are, therefore, needed.

Recent evidence suggesting that anti-chlamydial antibiotics may be of benefit in certain patients with established CHD needs to be confirmed by larger, purpose-designed, prospective trials (as highlighted in Chapter 6). Whether or not benefits of antibiotic therapy are limited to specific groups of patients with atherosclerotic disease also needs to be established.

Other issues to be resolved include: identification of any optimal antibiotic regimens and duration of therapy; the most appropriate means of monitoring *C. pneumoniae* infection status (including detection of reinfection); and whether the antibiotics are acting by independent, non-antimicrobial mechanisms as well as (or rather than) through anti-bacterial effects. It is equally important that widespread clinical use of broad-spectrum antibiotic therapy in the management of CHD does not occur prematurely. The indiscriminate use of broad-spectrum antibiotics in this context would raise concerns about potential related increases in the levels of bacterial resistance.[13] Evaluation of the risk–benefit balance of chronic antibiotic therapy in CHD patients is clearly essential.

The need to complete large-scale, randomised antibiotic intervention trials in patients with CHD is pressing. Further research is also needed to define clearly the direct role (if any) of *C. pneumoniae* in atherogenesis. In particular, whether there is a clear temporal relationship between acquisition of *C. pneumoniae* infection and CHD development, and how the infection might interact with conventional atherogenic risk factors, need clarification. The underlying mechanism of endothelial cell damage and/or plaque disruption (currently hypothesised to occur via macrophage activation) also requires further investigation. Such research could lead to increased understanding of CHD's pathogenesis and the development of new, effective management strategies over the next few years. The future development of a *C. pneumoniae* vaccine for potential use in the primary prevention of CHD may be a logical eventual development.

Chlamydia pneumoniae infection is common and treatable. If large-scale antibiotic intervention trials show conclusive long-term clinical benefit, antibiotic therapy may prove valuable in combating the 'epidemic' of CHD, which continues to be a major cause of morbidity and death worldwide. The potential implications for public health are obvious.

References

1. Gupta S. *Chlamydia pneumoniae*, monocyte activation and antimicrobial therapy in coronary heart disease. MD Thesis, 1999 (University of London, UK).
2. Saikku P, Mattila KJ, Nieminen MS *et al.* Serological evidence of an association of a novel chlamydia, TWAR, with chronic coronary heart disease and acute myocardial infarction. *Lancet* 1988; **ii**: 983–6.
3. Danesh J, Collins R, Peto R. Chronic infections and coronary heart disease: Is there a link? *Lancet* 1997; **350**: 430–6.
4. Gibbs RG and Davies AH. *Chlamydia pneumoniae* and vascular disease. *Br J Surg* 1998; **85**: 1191–7.
5. Ramirez JA. Isolation of *Chlamydia pneumoniae* from the coronary artery of a patient with coronary atherosclerosis. The *Chlamydia pneumoniae*/Atherosclerosis Study Group. *Ann Intern Med* 1996; **125**: 979–82.
6. Jackson LA, Campbell LA, Kuo CC *et al.* Isolation of *Chlamydia pneumoniae* from a carotid endarterectomy specimen. *J Infect Dis* 1997; **176**: 292–5.
7. Maass M, Bartels C, Engel PM, Mamut U, Sievens HH. Endovascular presence of viable *Chlamydia pneumoniae* is a common phenomenon in coronary artery disease. *J Am Coll Cardiol* 1998; **31**: 827–32.
8. Fong IW, Chiu B, Viira E *et al.* Rabbit models for *Chlamydia pneumoniae* infection. *J Clin Microbiol* 1997; **35**: 48–52.
9. Laitinen K, Laurila A, Pyhälä L, Leinonen M, Saikku P. *Chlamydia pneumoniae* infection induces inflammatory changes in the aortas of rabbits. *Infect Immun* 1997; **65**: 4832–5.
10. Muhlestein JB, Anderson JL, Hammond EH *et al.* Infection with *Chlamydia pneumoniae* accelerates the development of atherosclerosis and treatment with azithromycin prevents it in a rabbit model. *Circulation* 1998; **97**: 633–6.
11. Gupta S, Leatham EW, Carrington D *et al.* Elevated *Chlamydia pneumoniae* antibodies, cardiovascular events and azithromycin in male survivors of myocardial infarction. *Circulation* 1997; **96**: 404–17.
12. Gurfinkel E, Bozovich G, Darcoca A, Beck E, Mantner B. Randomised trial of roxithromycin in non-Q-wave coronary syndromes: ROXIS pilot study. *Lancet* 1997; **350**: 404–17.
13. Hart CA. Antibiotic resistance: an increasing problem? *BMJ* 1998; **316**: 1255–6.
14. Ånestad G, Scheel G, Hugnes O. Chronic infections and coronary heart disease. *Lancet* 1997, **350**: 1028 [letter].

Index

Developments in Cardiovascular Medicine

170. S.N. Willich and J.E. Muller (eds.): *Triggering of Acute Coronary Syndromes.* Implications for Prevention. 1995 ISBN 0-7923-3605-4
171. E.E. van der Wall, T.H. Marwick and J.H.C. Reiber (eds.): *Advances in Imaging Techniques in Ischemic Heart Disease.* 1995 ISBN 0-7923-3620-8
172. B. Swynghedauw: *Molecular Cardiology for the Cardiologist.* 1995 ISBN 0-7923-3622-4
173. C.A. Nienaber and U. Sechtem (eds.): *Imaging and Intervention in Cardiology.* 1996 ISBN 0-7923-3649-6
174. G. Assmann (ed.): *HDL Deficiency and Atherosclerosis.* 1995 ISBN 0-7923-8888-7
175. N.M. van Hemel, F.H.M. Wittkampf and H. Ector (eds.): *The Pacemaker Clinic of the 90's.* Essentials in Brady-Pacing. 1995 ISBN 0-7923-3688-7
176. N. Wilke (ed.): *Advanced Cardiovascular MRI of the Heart and Great Vessels.* Forthcoming. ISBN 0-7923-3720-4
177. M. LeWinter, H. Suga and M.W. Watkins (eds.): *Cardiac Energetics: From Emax to Pressure-volume Area.* 1995 ISBN 0-7923-3721-2
178. R.J. Siegel (ed.): *Ultrasound Angioplasty.* 1995 ISBN 0-7923-3722-0
179. D.M. Yellon and G.J. Gross (eds.): *Myocardial Protection and the K_{ATP} Channel.* 1995 ISBN 0-7923-3791-3
180. A.V.G. Bruschke, J.H.C. Reiber, K.I. Lie and H.J.J. Wellens (eds.): *Lipid Lowering Therapy and Progression of Coronary Atherosclerosis.* 1996 ISBN 0-7923-3807-3
181. A.-S.A. Abd-Eyattah and A.S. Wechsler (eds.): *Purines and Myocardial Protection.* 1995 ISBN 0-7923-3831-6
182. M. Morad, S. Ebashi, W. Trautwein and Y. Kurachi (eds.): *Molecular Physiology and Pharmacology of Cardiac Ion Channels and Transporters.* 1996 ISBN 0-7923-3913-4
183. M.A. Oto (ed.): *Practice and Progress in Cardiac Pacing and Electrophysiology.* 1996 ISBN 0-7923-3950-9
184. W.H. Birkenhäger (ed.): *Practical Management of Hypertension.* Second Edition. 1996 ISBN 0-7923-3952-5
185. J.C. Chatham, J.R. Forder and J.H. McNeill (eds.): *The Heart in Diabetes.* 1996 ISBN 0-7923-4052-3
186. J.H.C. Reiber and E.E. van der Wall (eds.): *Cardiovascular Imaging.* 1996 ISBN 0-7923-4109-0
187. A-M. Salmasi and A. Strano (eds.): *Angiology in Practice.* 1996 ISBN 0-7923-4143-0
188. M.W. Kroll and M.H. Lehmann (eds.): *Implantable Cardioverter Defibrillator Therapy: The Engineering – Clinical Interface.* 1996 ISBN 0-7923-4300-X
189. K.L. March (ed.): *Gene Transfer in the Cardiovascular System.* Experimental Approaches and Therapeutic Implications. 1996 ISBN 0-7923-9859-9
190. L. Klein (ed.): *Coronary Stenosis Morphology: Analysis and Implication.* 1997 ISBN 0-7923-9867-X
191. J.E. Pérez and R.M. Lang (eds.): *Echocardiography and Cardiovascular Function: Tools for the Next Decade.* 1997 ISBN 0-7923-9884-X
192. A.A. Knowlton (ed.): *Heat Shock Proteins and the Cardiovascular System.* 1997 ISBN 0-7923-9910-2
193. R.C. Becker (ed.): *The Textbook of Coronary Thrombosis and Thrombolysis.* 1997 ISBN 0-7923-9923-4
194. R.M. Mentzer, Jr., M. Kitakaze, J.M. Downey and M. Hori (eds.): *Adenosine, Cardioprotection and Its Clinical Application.* 1997 ISBN 0-7923-9954-4
195. N.H.J. Pijls and B. De Bruyne: *Coronary Pressure.* 1997 ISBN 0-7923-4672-6
196. I. Graham, H. Refsum, I.H. Rosenberg and P.M. Ueland (eds.): *Homocysteine Metabolism: from Basic Science to Clinical Medicine.* 1997 ISBN 0-7923-9983-8
197. E.E. van der Wall, V. Manger Cats and J. Baan (eds.): *Vascular Medicine – From Endothelium to Myocardium.* 1997 ISBN 0-7923-4740-4
198. A. Lafont and E. Topol (eds.): *Arterial Remodeling.* A Critical Factor in Restenosis. 1997 ISBN 0-7923-8008-8
199. M. Mercury, D.D. McPherson, H. Bassiouny and S. Glagov (eds.): *Non-Invasive Imaging of Atherosclerosis* 1998 ISBN 0-7923-8036-3
200. W.C. De Mello and M.J. Janse (eds.): *Heart Cell Communication in Health and Disease.* 1997 ISBN 0-7923-8052-5

Developments in Cardiovascular Medicine

201. P.E. Vardas (ed.): *Cardiac Arrhythmias Pacing and Electrophysiology.* The Expert View. 1998 ISBN 0-7923-4908-3
202. E.E. van der Wall, P.K. Blanksma, M.G. Niemeyer, W. Vaalburg and H.J.G.M. Crijns (eds.): *Advanced Imaging in Coronary Artery Disease.* PET, SPECT, MRI, IVUS, EBCT. 1998 ISBN 0-7923-5083-9
203. R.L. Wilenski (ed.): *Unstable Coronary Artery Syndromes, Pathophysiology, Diagnosis and Treatment.* 1998 ISBN 0-7923-8201-3
204. J.H.C. Reiber and E.E. van der Wall (eds.): *What's New in Cardiovascular Imaging?* 1998 ISBN 0-7923-5121-5
205. J.C. Kaski and D.W. Holt (eds.): *Myocardial Damage.* Early Detection by Novel Biochemical Markers. 1998 ISBN 0-7923-5140-1
206. M. Malik (ed.): *Clinical Guide to Cardiac Autonomic Tests.* 1998 ISBN 0-7923-5178-9
207. G.F. Baxter and D.M. Yellon (eds.): *Delayed Preconditioning and Adaptive Cardioprotection.* 1998 ISBN 0-7923-5259-9
208. B. Swynghedauw, *Molecular Cardiology for the Cardiologist, Second Edition.* 1998 ISBN 0-7923-8323-0
209. G. Burnstock, J.G. Dobson, Jr., B.T. Liang, J. Linden (eds.): *Cardiovascular Biology of Purines.* 1998 ISBN 0-7923-8334-6
210. B.D. Hoit, R.A. Walsh (eds.): *Cardiovascular Physiology in the Genetically Engineered Mouse.* 1998 ISBN 0-7923-8356-7
211. P. Whittaker, G.S. Abela (eds.): *Direct Myocardial Revascularization: History, Methodology, Technology.* 1998 ISBN 0-7923-8398-2
212. C.A. Nienaber and R. Fattori (eds.): *Diagnosis and Treatment of Aortic Diseases.* 1999 ISBN 0-7923-5517-2
213. J.C. Kaski (ed.): *Chest Pain with Normal Coronary Angiograms: Pathogenesis, Diagnosis and Management.* 1999 ISBN 0-7923-8421-0
214. P.A. Doevendans, R.S. Reneman and M. van Bilsen (eds.): *Cardiovascular Specific Gene Expression.* 1999 ISBN 0-7923-5633-0
215. G. Pons-Lladó, F. Carreras, X. Borrás, M. Subirana and L.J. Jiménez-Borreguero (eds.): *Atlas of Practical Cardiac Applications of MRI.* 1999 ISBN 0-7923-5636-5
216. L.W. Klein and J.E. Calvin, *Resource Ultilization in Cardiac Disease.* 1999 ISBN 0-7923-8509-8
217. R. Gorlin, G. Dangas, P.K. Toutouzas and M.M. Konstadoulaks: *Contemporary Concepts in Cardiology, Pathophysiology and Clinical Management.* 1999 ISBN 0-7923-8514-4
218. S. Gupta and A.J. Camm: *Chronic Infection, Chlamydia and Coronary Heart Disease.* 1999 ISBN 0-7923-5797-3
219. M. Rajskina: *Ventricular Fibrillation in Sudden Cardiac Death.* 1999 ISBN 0-7923-8570-5
220. Z. Abedin and R. Conner: *Interpretation of Cardiac Arrhythmias: Self Assessment Approach.* 1999 ISBN 0-7923-8576-4
221. J.E. Lock, J.F. Keane and S.B. Perry (eds.): *Diagnostic and Interventional Catheterization in Congenital Heart Disease, second edition.* 1999 ISBN 0-7923-8597-7

Previous volumes are still available

KLUWER ACADEMIC PUBLISHERS – DORDRECHT / BOSTON / LONDON